Dental Sleep Medicine

Editor

JAMISON R. SPENCER

SLEEP MEDICINE CLINICS

www.sleep.theclinics.com

Consulting Editor
TEOFILO LEE-CHIONG Jr

December 2018 • Volume 13 • Number 4

ELSEVIER

1600 John F. Kennedy Boulevard • Suite 1800 • Philadelphia, Pennsylvania, 19103-2899

http://www.theclinics.com

SLEEP MEDICINE CLINICS Volume 13, Number 4
December 2018, ISSN 1556-407X, ISBN-13: 978-0-323-64334-4

Editor: Colleen Dietzler
Developmental Editor: Donald Mumford

Sleep Medicine Clinics (ISSN 1556-407X) is published quarterly by Elsevier Inc., 360 Park Avenue South, New York, NY 10010-1710. Months of issue are March, June, September and December. Business and Editorial Offices: 1600 John F. Kennedy Blvd., Ste. 1800, Philadelphia, PA 19103-2899. Customer Service Office: 3251 Riverport Lane, Maryland Heights, MO 63043. Periodicals postage paid at New York, NY and additional mailing offices. Subscription prices are $203.00 per year (US individuals), $100.00 (US students), $486.00 (US institutions), $245.00 (Canadian and international individuals), $135.00 (Canadian and international students), $540.00 (Canadian institutions) and $540.00 (International institutions). Foreign air speed delivery is included in all *Clinics* subscription prices. All prices are subject to change without notice. **POSTMASTER:** Send change of address to *Sleep Medicine Clinics*, Elsevier Health Sciences Division, Subscription Customer Service, 3251 Riverport Lane, Maryland Heights, MO 63043. Customer Service: **Tel: 1-800-654-2452 (U.S. and Canada); 314-447-8871 (outside U.S. and Canada). Fax: 314-447-8029. E-mail: journalscustomerservice-usa@elsevier.com (for print support); journalsonline support-usa@elsevier.com (for online support).**

Reprints. For copies of 100 or more of articles in this publication, please contact the Commercial Reprints Department, Elsevier Inc., 360 Park Avenue South, New York, NY 10010-1710. Tel.: 212-633-3874; Fax: 212-633-3820; E-mail: reprints@elsevier.com.

Sleep Medicine Clinics is covered in *MEDLINE/PubMed (Index Medicus)*.

PROGRAM OBJECTIVE

The goal of *Sleep Clinics of North America* is to keep practicing physicians up to date with current clinical practice by providing timely articles reviewing the state of the art in patient care.

TARGET AUDIENCE

All practicing physicians and other healthcare professionals.

LEARNING OBJECTIVES

Upon completion of this activity, participants will be able to:

1. Review potential side effects and clinical guidelines for oral appliance therapy in the treatment of obstructive sleep apnea.
2. Discuss the role dentists have in identifying and assisting with the management of Pediatric obstructive sleep apnea.
3. Recognize the use of transcranial magnetic stimulation in dental sleep medicine, its mechanisms and applications to obstructive sleep apnea and sleep bruxism

ACCREDITATION

The Elsevier Office of Continuing Medical Education (EOCME) is accredited by the Accreditation Council for Continuing Medical Education (ACCME) to provide continuing medical education for physicians.

The EOCME designates this enduring material for a maximum of 15 *AMA PRA Category 1 Credit*(s)™. Physicians should claim only the credit commensurate with the extent of their participation in the activity.

All other healthcare professionals requesting continuing education credit for this enduring material will be issued a certificate of participation.

DISCLOSURE OF CONFLICTS OF INTEREST

The EOCME assesses conflict of interest with its instructors, faculty, planners, and other individuals who are in a position to control the content of CME activities. All relevant conflicts of interest that are identified are thoroughly vetted by EOCME for fair balance, scientific objectivity, and patient care recommendations. EOCME is committed to providing its learners with CME activities that promote improvements or quality in healthcare and not a specific proprietary business or a commercial interest.

The planning committee, staff, authors and editors listed below have identified no financial relationships or relationships to products or devices they or their spouse/life partner have with commercial interest related to the content of this CME activity:

Herrero Babiloni A, DDS, MS; José E. Barrera, MD, FACS; Scott B. Boyd, DDS, PhD; Macario Camacho, MAJ, MD; Leopoldo P. Correa, BDS, MS; Raj Daniels, MAJ, MD; Louis De Beaumont, PhD; B. Gail Demko, DMD; Carolyn C. Dicus Brookes, DMD, MD; Colleen Dietzier; Alison Kemp; Cameron A. Kuehne, DMD, MS; Gilles J. Lavigne, DMD, PhD, FRCD; Teofilo Lee-Chiong Jr, MD; Noshir R. Mehta, BDS, DMD, MS; Manuel Pozo-Alonso, COL, DDS; Arunkumar Rangarajan; Thomas G. Schell, DMD, DABDSM; Jamison R. Spencer, DMD, MS; Thomas R. Stark, LTC, DDS.

The planning committee, staff, authors and editors listed below have identified financial relationships or relationships to products or devices they or their spouse/life partner have with commercial interest related to the content of this CME activity:

Steve Carstensen, DDS, FAGD, FACD, FICD, DABDSM: *is a consultant/advisor for Sleep Architects, Inc.*

UNAPPROVED/OFF-LABEL USE DISCLOSURE

The EOCME requires CME faculty to disclose to the participants:

1. When products or procedures being discussed are off-label, unlabelled, experimental, and/or investigational (not US Food and Drug Administration [FDA] approved); and
2. Any limitations on the information presented, such as data that are preliminary or that represent ongoing research, interim analyses, and/or unsupported opinions. Faculty may discuss information about pharmaceutical agents that is outside of FDA-approved labelling. This information is intended solely for CME and is not intended to promote off-label use of these medications. If you have any questions, contact the medical affairs department of the manufacturer for the most recent prescribing information.

TO ENROLL

To enroll in the *Sleep Medicines Clinic* Continuing Medical Education program, call customer service at 1-800-654-2452 or sign up online at http://www.theclinics.com/home/cme. The CME program is available to subscribers for an additional annual fee of USD $140.

METHOD OF PARTICIPATION

In order to claim credit, participants must complete the following:

1. Complete enrolment as indicated above.
2. Read the activity.

3. Complete the CME Test and Evaluation. Participants must achieve a score of 70% on the test. All CME Tests and Evaluations must be completed online.

CME INQUIRIES/SPECIAL NEEDS
For all CME inquiries or special needs, please contact elsevierCME@elsevier.com.

SLEEP MEDICINE CLINICS

THE CLINICS ARE AVAILABLE ONLINE!
Access your subscription at:
www.theclinics.com

Contributors

CONSULTING EDITOR

TEOFILO LEE-CHIONG Jr, MD
Professor of Medicine, National Jewish Health,
University of Colorado Denver, Denver,
Colorado, USA; Chief Medical Liaison, Philips
Respironics, Pennsylvania, USA

EDITOR

JAMISON R. SPENCER, DMD, MS
The Center for Sleep Apnea and TMJ, Salt Lake
City, Utah, USA; Adjunct Faculty, University of
the Pacific Arthur A. Dugoni School of
Dentistry, Adjunct Faculty, University of
North Carolina at Chapel Hill School of
Dentistry, North Carolina, USA

AUTHORS

HERRERO BABILONI A, DDS, MS
Center for Advanced Research in Sleep
Medicine, Hôpital Du Sacre-Coeur, CIUSSS
Nord Ile Montréal, Université De Montréal,
Montréal, Québec, Canada

JOSÉ E. BARRERA, MD, FACS
Associate Professor, Department of Surgery,
Uniformed Services University, Bethesda,
Maryland, USA; Clinical Associate Professor,
Department of Otolaryngology, The University
of Texas Health Sciences Center, Medical
Director, Texas Facial Plastic Surgery and ENT,
San Antonio, Texas, USA

SCOTT B. BOYD, DDS, PhD
Professor, Oral and Maxillofacial Surgery,
Retired, Vanderbilt University School of
Medicine, Nashville, Tennessee, USA

MACARIO CAMACHO, MAJ, MD
Assistant Professor, Uniformed Service Health
Science University, Division of Otolaryngology–
Head and Neck Surgery, Tripler Army Medical
Center, Honolulu, Hawaii, USA

**STEVE CARSTENSEN, DDS, FAGD, FACD,
FICD, DABDSM**
Private Practice, Premier Sleep Associates,
Bellevue, Washington, USA; Editor in Chief,
Dental Sleep Practice Magazine; Sleep
Education Director, The Pankey Institute,
Key Biscayne, Florida, USA; Adjunct Visiting
Faculty, Louisiana State University Dental
School, New Orleans, Louisiana, USA; Guest
Lecturer, The University of the Pacific, San
Francisco, California, USA; Guest Lecturer,
Spear Education, Scottsdale, Arizona, USA

LEOPOLDO P. CORREA, BDS, MS
Director, Dental Sleep Medicine Fellowship
Program, Division of Craniofacial Pain Center,
Associate Professor, Department of Diagnostic
Sciences, Tufts University School of Dental
Medicine, Boston, Massachusetts, USA

RAJ DANIELS, MAJ, MD
Instructor of Pediatrics, Uniformed Service
Health Science University, Department of
Pediatrics, Division of Sleep Medicine, Tripler
Army Medical Center, Honolulu, Hawaii, USA

LOUIS DE BEAUMONT, PhD
Center for Advanced Research in Sleep
Medicine, Hôpital Du Sacre-Coeur, CIUSSS
Nord Ile Montréal, Université De Montréal,
Montréal, Québec, Canada

B. GAIL DEMKO, DMD
Education Director, Sleep Apnea Dentists
of New England, Newton, Massachusetts, USA

CAROLYN C. DICUS BROOKES, DMD, MD
Assistant Professor, Interim Division
Chief, Division of Oral and Maxillofacial
Surgery, Froedtert & the Medical College
of Wisconsin, Milwaukee, Wisconsin, USA

CAMERON A. KUEHNE, DMD, MS
Pacific Dugoni School of Dentistry,
San Francisco, California, USA; American
Academy of Dental Sleep Medicine Mastery
Program, Lisle, Illinois, USA; American
Academy of Craniofacial Pain Institute, Reston,
Virginia, Co-Owner, The Center for Sleep
Apnea and TMJ, Boise, Idaho, USA

GILLES J. LAVIGNE, DMD, PhD, FRCD
Center for Advanced Research in Sleep
Medicine, Hôpital Du Sacre-Coeur, CIUSSS
Nord Ile Montréal, Université De Montréal,
Montréal, Québec, Canada

NOSHIR R. MEHTA, BDS, DMD, MS
Professor and Associate Dean for Global
Relations, Department of Public Health, Past
Director and Current Senior Consultant,
Craniofacial Pain and Sleep Center, Tufts
University School of Dental Medicine,
Boston, Massachusetts, USA

MANUEL POZO-ALONSO, COL, DDS
Assistant Professor, Uniformed Service
Health Science University, Department
of Orthodontics, Dental Health
Activity Rheinland Pfalz, Landstuhl,
Germany

THOMAS G. SCHELL, DMD, DABDSM
Owner, Dr. Thomas G Schell and Dr. Patrick C
Noble PLLC, Lebanon, New Hampshire, USA;
Adjunctive Administrative Assistant Professor,
Department of Surgery, Dartmouth Geisel
School of Medicine, Hanover, New Hampshire,
USA

THOMAS R. STARK, LTC, DDS
Assistant Professor, Uniformed Service Health
Science University, Departments of Pediatric
Dentistry and Orofacial Pain, Dental Health
Activity Rheinland Pfalz, Wiesbaden,
Germany

Contents

and management of common side effects, and adhere to current standards of dental sleep medicine practice.

Adding airway services to a dental practice disrupts scheduling, examinations, treatment planning, billing, and team roles. Problems connected with the airway can be addressed with more precise therapy and better prognosis while building confidence between the patient and the dental team. Each team member must understand the connections between airway problems and patient health and be able to talk about it with confidence. If the entire team supports the inclusion of airway therapy into the service mix, patients will feel well cared for and rewards to the office will be plentiful.

Pediatric obstructive sleep apnea (OSA) is a serious medical condition with numerous health consequences. Dentists are well suited to recognize and provide medical referrals for pediatric patients at risk for OSA. Timely dental sleep medicine interventions may improve signs and symptoms of OSA in growing children. Orthodontic and dentofacial orthopedic treatment may decrease obstructive respiratory events in some pediatric patients. Palatal expansion may be part of a comprehensive orthodontic treatment plan to correct a malocclusion and treat OSA. Orthognathic surgery, mandibular advancement devices, and oropharyngeal exercises may have a role in the management of OSA in pediatric and adolescent patients.

Multilevel surgery has been established as the mainstay of treatment for the surgical management of obstructive sleep apnea (OSA). Combined with uvulopalatopharyngoplasty, tongue-base surgeries, including the genioglossus advancement (GA), sliding genioplasty, and hyoid myotomy and suspension, have been developed to target hypopharyngeal obstruction. Total airway surgery consisting of maxillomandibular advancement (MMA) with/without GA has shown significant success. Skeletal procedures for OSA with or without a palatal procedure is a proven technique for relieving airway obstruction during sleep. A case study demonstrating the utility of virtual surgical planning for MMA surgery is presented.

Obstructive sleep apnea (OSA) is a common chronic disease characterized by repetitive pharyngeal collapse during sleep. OSA is associated with cardiovascular disease and increased mortality, among other issues. Continuous positive airway pressure (CPAP) is considered first-line therapy for OSA, but is not always tolerated. Both nonsurgical and surgical alternative management strategies are available for the CPAP-intolerant patient. This article explores controversies surrounding airway evaluation, definition of successful treatment, and surgical management of the

CPAP-intolerant patient with moderate to severe OSA. Controversies specific to maxillomandibular advancement also are discussed.

Transcranial Magnetic Stimulation: Potential Use in Obstructive Sleep Apnea and Sleep Bruxism

Herrero Babiloni A, Louis De Beaumont, and Gilles J. Lavigne

The aim of this article is to introduce transcranial magnetic stimulation (TMS) to dental practitioners and to explain its use in obstructive sleep apnea (OSA) and sleep bruxism (SB). In these 2 sleep disorders, TMS has proven to be a useful tool to explore pathophysiological pathways and disease mechanisms, and in a more limited way, to recruit upper airway muscles in OSA and reduce muscle activity and pain intensity in SB. Although promising, research using TMS in these conditions is still very limited and future investigations should be conducted before its clinical application can be considered.

Contents

The aim of this article is to introduce transcranial magnetic stimulation (TMS) to dental practitioners and to explain its use in obstructive sleep apnea (OSA) and sleep bruxism (SB). In these 2 sleep disorders, TMS has proven to be a useful tool to explore pathophysiological pathways and disease mechanisms, and in a more limited way, to recruit upper airway muscles in OSA and reduce muscle activity and pain intensity in SB. Although promising, research using TMS in these conditions is still very limited and future investigations should be conducted before its clinical application can be considered.

Preface

Beyond Blowing: Oral Appliance Therapy, Surgery, and Transcranial Magnetic Stimulation

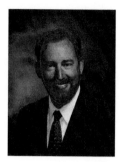

Jamison R. Spencer, DMD, MS
Editor

It has been my pleasure to act as editor of this issue of *Sleep Medicine Clinics.*

Not everyone can tolerate positive airway pressure (PAP) therapy. And PAP isn't always the best therapeutic option for the obstructive sleep apnea (OSA) patient.

Oral appliance therapy and surgical approaches in the treatment of OSA have been around for a very long time and have provided alternative, and sometimes adjunctive, options for our patients.

If you are a physician, you may have heard that oral appliance therapy is only for mild cases and causes TMJ problems, bite changes, and other problems. Physicians and dentists alike may have heard that surgery in general is ineffective and only bimaxillary advancement (also known as orthognathic surgery) works (other than tracheostomy, of course). In this issue, we address these areas of potential concern and controversy.

For physicians reading this, I hope it provides you with a good overview of options that are available to your OSA patients that you may be less familiar with, as well as providing a window into the world of those who dedicate their professional careers to providing these therapies and procedures. You'll learn that qualified dentists well trained in the care of patients with OSA go far beyond "just fitting a piece of plastic," and that the preparatory work going into skeletal surgery is as critical to success as the surgical procedure itself.

For dentists reading this, you will be able to learn everything from the history of oral appliance therapy to the latest techniques, procedures, and protocols from initial screening to final follow-up. This publication may be used as a helpful guide and reference in your evaluation and treatment of both adults and children as well as help you better understand the surgical approaches from which many of your patients may benefit.

To all who take the time to review this issue, I am confident that you will be rewarded with a deeper understanding of nonsurgical and surgical approaches that are available to help the patients you serve. As physicians, dentists, and other health care providers work together through the screening, diagnosis, and treatment process, our patients are the ones who will benefit from better, more predictable, and more effective outcomes.

Jamison R. Spencer, DMD, MS
The Center for Sleep Apnea and TMJ
Redwood Dental Specialty Plaza
6287 South Redwood Road, Suite 101
Salt Lake City, UT 84123, USA

E-mail address:
Jamison@JamisonSpencer.com

Sleep Med Clin 13 (2018) xiii
https://doi.org/10.1016/j.jsmc.2018.09.001
1556-407X/18/© 2018 Published by Elsevier Inc.

sleep.theclinics.com

The Evolution of Oral Appliance Therapy for Snoring and Sleep Apnea
Where Did We Come From, Where Are We, and Where Are We Going?

B. Gail Demko, DMD

KEYWORDS

- Oral appliance history • Von Esmarch • Jaw thrust • Phenotype • Titration

KEY POINTS

- Oral appliance therapy (OAT) for the treatment of snoring and obstructive sleep apnea is accepted as the most effective noninvasive therapy second only to continuous positive airway pressure.
- This article explains the innovations of the previous 200 years and how they laid the groundwork for OAT today.
- The expansion of this treatment over the past 40 years has been explosive and evidence based.
- The future will be linked to changes in the medical field, continued research on appliance design, and development of personalized medicine that will appropriately identify therapy options.

INTRODUCTION

Oral appliance therapy has long existed within the purview of dental therapy. With the advent of the field of sleep medicine, dentists were able to add their skills and knowledge to that of physicians in the treatment of patients with sleep-disordered breathing, predominantly snoring and obstructive sleep apnea (OSA). But where did this area of knowledge originate? What knowledge was required to apply oral appliance therapy to the nascent field of sleep medicine? It did not spring like Aphrodite from the foam of the sea, but from a vast network of knowledge and beliefs that preceded our present understanding of oral appliance therapy (OAT) by more than a century. This included 3 things: a cultural belief that there was healthy breathing and unhealthy breathing, medical acceptance that mechanical means could keep the airway open and, finally, an understanding that there were people who suffered from interrupted breathing at night. This article elucidates some of the steps that paved the way for the present field of dental sleep medicine. It is logically within the purview of medicine to give dentists the information they need to successfully treat patients and it is within the purview of dentistry to identify appropriate appliance designs and provide ongoing care for those who suffer from snoring and OSA. Going forward, the fields of sleep medicine and dental sleep medicine must continue to advance together to provide appropriate therapy for those who suffer. This article discusses dentistry's role in treating this burgeoning medical problem.

EARLY HISTORY, 1860 TO 1980: BUILDING BLOCKS LEADING TO ORAL APPLIANCE THERAPY
Cultural Knowledge

During this 120-year period, all the building blocks of OAT for the treatment of OSA were laid. In 1861, the ethnographer George Catlin first published his treatise entitled "The Breath of Life or mal-respiration

Sleep Apnea Dentists of New England, 70 Wells Avenue, Newton, MA 02459 USA
E-mail address: drdemko@sleepapneadentist.com

Sleep Med Clin 13 (2018) 467–487
https://doi.org/10.1016/j.jsmc.2018.07.001
1556-407X/18/Published by Elsevier Inc.

and its effects upon the enjoyments and life of man."[1] He based his thoughts on decades of travel among Native American peoples in both North and South America. Catlin became convinced that, before the introduction of alcohol, the robust health of native races was due to "quiet and natural sleep...The air which enters the mouth is as different from that which enters the nostrils as distilled water is different from the water in... a frog pond."[1(p24)] He blamed all evils of modern men on sleeping with an open mouth. He stressed that the nose was made to filter "infinitesimal insects, poisonous minerals and poisonous effluvia" and a closed mouth existence led to straight healthy teeth while preventing epidemic diseases such as cholera and yellow fever.[1(p30)] Published under various titles over the next 30 years, the idea that nasal breathing was healthy breathing became a widespread belief throughout the English-speaking world.

Medical Knowledge

Medicine has long shared information via journals and publications, thus it is very difficult to pinpoint the exact nascence of any specific idea. All ideas are based on prior knowledge and prior learning filtered through cultural beliefs, lectures, journals, texts, and visiting professors. We accept that general anesthesia came into use in the early 1840s, and much was written about its dangers, including the "stoppage of the passage of air" and that "to deal with the partial obstruction...the mere depressing or raising of the chin was enough to close or open the passage."[2] Airway obstruction, related to general anesthesia, was dealt with widely, not only by doing a head tilt, but holding the tongue forward out of the oral cavity with forceps or doing a jaw thrust maneuver. These latter 2 techniques reached a worldwide audience when the German military surgeon, Frederick von Esmarch (1823–1908), published his massive *Handbook of Surgery*,[3] which represented his then modern views of military surgery. In the section on chloroform anesthesia, von Esmarch explains how to manage a patient who developed closure of the upper airway during a surgical procedure. In one scenario, he writes that the glottis may close by "spasm of the muscles of the larynx and tongue. Prompt action is now imperative to free the upper entrance to the larynx. The jaws must be separated, the tongue must be drawn well out of the mouth"[3(p116)] (**Fig. 1**). von Esmarch credited a second scenario to prevent asphyxia to British surgeon, J.S. Little,[4] who visited Kiel, Germany, in 1866. This maneuver required the

surgeon, positioned behind the patient, to lift the lower jaw, "apply both hands to the neck in such a manner that the forefingers come to lie behind the ascending rami of the lower maxilla [mandible]; push the whole lower jaw forward until the lower row of teeth projects beyond the upper [subluxation]"[3(p115)] (**Fig. 2**). This information spread around the world with multiple foreign language translations of von Esmarch's text, including English editions in both 1897 and 1901. It is probable that both medical and dental practitioners came in contact with these ideas during their training.[a] The concept of tongue extension and a jaw thrust maneuver are the basis behind all present-day medically accepted OA.

The First Real Step

In January 1923, Pierre Robin[5] (1867–1950), a French physician and dentist, who practiced in the Children's Hospital in Paris, presented a case to the Academy of Medicine about a new cause that prevented pure nasal breathing due to the "relapse of the base of the tongue pressing on the epiglottis and closing the ...opening of the larynx"; he called this "glossoptosis." Robin came upon this "discovery" after realizing that adenoidectomy was not always successful in establishing nasal breathing and, therefore, there must be another cause for mouth breathing. "It [airway obstruction] disappears immediately as soon as the subject extends his jaw to the front and keeps his lips open" and "[t]his form of airway obstruction [is] easily distinguished from naso-pharyngeal respiratory obstruction by asking the patient to "extend his lower mandible forward and up in such a way that his lower incisors are further forward than his upper ones.... Essential glossoptosis can easily be suppressed by moving the chin forward, thereby advancing the entire floor of the mouth, the tongue and the musculature which attaches to the lower jaw and the hyoid bone." Robin placed a mono-block (one-piece) oral appliance (OA) and suggested that it be worn continuously, with changes dictated by growth and development, from ages 3 to 18, thus presaging the use of orthodontic devices for the treatment of OSA in the 1980s.

Tools to Work with

Emil Herbst (1872–1940), a German orthodontist, presented on the use of his Herbst appliance in 1909 at the Fifth International Dental Congress in Berlin; it was a fixed appliance designed for correction of skeletal Class II malocclusions. The Herbst appliance fell into obscurity after 1934 until it was "rediscovered" in the late 1970s by Hans Pancherz,

---

[a]The technique of a jaw thrust continues to be called the Esmarch maneuver in Germany.

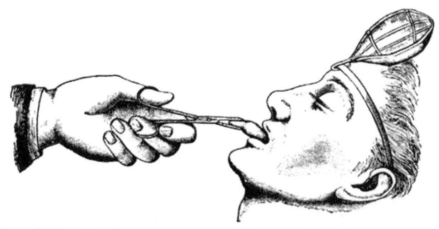

Fig. 1. von Esmarch's illustration of tongue extension for maintenance of the airway if respiration declines during chloroform anesthesia, 1877. (*From* Esmarch F. Handbuch der Kriegschirurgischen Technik. Eine gekrönte Preisschrift. Hannover (Germany): Carl Rűmpler; 1877. p. 112–25.)

DDS,[6] a German orthodontist. Howe and McNamara[7–9] redesigned the fixed Herbst into a removable acrylic splint in the 1980s,[9] coincident with the early phase of OA therapy for snoring and OSA. This device, with telescoping articulated arms, is now 1 of only 2 styles of appliance approved by Medicare for the treatment of OSA.

RECENT HISTORY, 1890 TO 1970: ORAL APPLIANCES USED TO PREVENT SNORING OR MAINTAIN AN OPEN AIRWAY

By 1984, it was reported that the US Patent Office had granted more than 300 patents for devices purported to stop snoring.[10] Although most of these were extraoral, for example, chinstraps (1891)[11] or nasal dilators (1918),[12] intraoral devices were also patented. These included mouth shields developed to force nasal breathing (1903)[13] or a

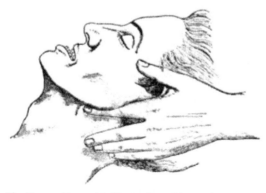

Fig. 2. von Esmarch's illustration of jaw advancement for maintenance of the airway if respiration declines during chloroform anesthesia 1877. (*From* Esmarch F. Handbuch der Kriegschirurgischen Technik. Eine gekrönte Preisschrift. Hannover (Germany): Carl Rűmpler; 1877. p. 112–25.)

gag-style device (1897)[14] to prevent tongue displacement and allow oral breathing. In 1927, Edward J. King[15] received patent no. 1674336 for a "respirator" that was meant "for placement between the teeth of the user for preventing snoring and for facilitating breathing" (**Fig. 3**). A device for constraining the tongue was patented in 1958 to prevent the tongue from falling back so as to "partially or completely block the tracheal passage…so as to cause suffocation"; the soft-palate lifter was patented by Corniello in 1964.[16] Creative measures all, but none of them found success in the treatment of OSA.

The knowledge base for dental sleep medicine (DSM) was now in the public domain, thanks to the popular press, medical journals, and texts. This coalesced with the use of OAs both within the dental profession and by erstwhile inventors, ripe for medical advancement that defined the disease of OSA in the 1970s.

SEMINAL HISTORY, 1970 TO 1985: THE TIPPING POINT
Medical Advances

Though Richard Caton (1842–1926) wrote of an obese poultry dealer who fell asleep while waiting on customers in 1889, he erroneously termed this a case of narcolepsy.[17] He described the patient's breathing during sleep as "a spasmodic closure of the glottis entirely suspending respiration…once yielding, a series of long inspirations and expirations follows." The president of the medical society, Christopher Heath, alluded to the resemblance of the poultry dealer to Joe, the sleepy boy in Dickens' *The Posthumous Papers of the Pickwick Club* first published in 1837.[18] Pickwickian syndrome was thought to be a problem of obese people falling

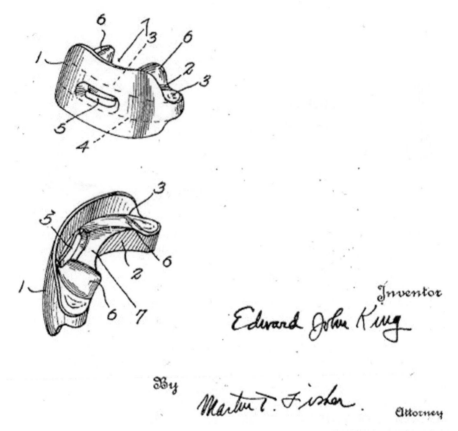

Fig. 3. Patent application drawings of a "Respirator" by Edward John King, 1927. (*From* King EG. US patent application for oral 'respirator'. 1927. Available at: http://pdfpiw.uspto.gov/.piw?Docid=01674336&homeurl=http%3A%2F%2Fpatft.uspto.gov%2Fnetacgi%2Fnph-Parser%3FSect1%3DPTO1%2526Sect2%3DHITOFF%2526d%3DPALL%2526p%3D1%2526u%3D%25252Fnetahtml%25252FPTO%25252Fsrchnum.htm%2526r%3D1%2526f%3DG%2526l%3D50%2526s1%3D1674336.PN.%2526OS%3DPN%2F1674336%2526RS%3DPN%2F1674336&PageNum=&Rtype=&SectionNum=&idkey=NONE&Input=View+first+page. Accessed December 12, 2017.)

asleep during the day. Not until 1964, when German neurologist Wolfgang Kuhl[19] did nighttime electroencephalogram recordings, was it found that the real cause of the problem was frequent arousals from sleep. In 1973, Guilleminault and colleagues[20] published their seminal paper in *Science*, in which they described disrupted sleep breathing in patients who were not obese; this was the first description of sleep apnea syndrome. The pathophysiology of this syndrome was elucidated by Remmers and colleagues[21] in 1978. Treatment with weight loss was infrequently effective, and tracheostomy serendipitously became the treatment of choice in approximately 1970.[22] It was of great interest, then, in 1981 when Colin Sullivan and colleagues[23] published in *Lancet* that nasal continuous positive airway pressure (CPAP) could reverse OSA. Years of research has led to positive airway pressure (PAP) being considered the "gold standard" of therapy for OSA.

Early Oral Appliance Therapy: The Pioneers

At the same time that Sullivan and colleagues[23] reported the concept of PAP in *Lancet*, a Chicago psychiatrist, Charles F. Samelson (1917–1999), motivated by his own snoring problem, developed a wax "tongue sleeve" to hold his tongue forward during sleep. This echoes the writings of von Esmarch and others who wrote about the dangers of chloroform anesthesia 100 years earlier. This tongue retaining device (TRD) prevented mouth breathing and physically held the tongue forward and partially outside the oral cavity, increasing the size of the oropharynx. Because the wax was brittle and broke frequently, the TRD, patented as an antisnoring/antibruxism appliance in 1979,[24] was made out of the synthetic plastic (copolymer) resin ethylene vinyl acetate. Repatented in 1981, the purpose of the TRD was expanded to include "avoidance of obstructive sleep apnea" (**Fig. 4**). Dr Samelson took his TRD to Rosalind D. Cartwright,

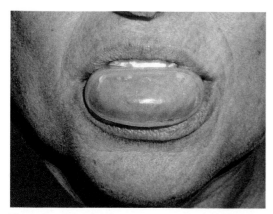

Fig. 4. A custom-made tongue retaining device (TRD) designed by Charles F. Samelson, MD. (*Courtesy of* Kelly Doyle, KDNight Laboratory, Racine, WI; with permission.)

PhD, and their first clinical trial, which showed comparable clinical outcome to uvulopalatopharyngoplasty (UPPP), was published in *JAMA* in 1982.[25]

Meanwhile, in Germany, a neurologist and sleep physician, Karlheinz Meier-Ewert read the *JAMA* article by Cartwright and Samelson[25] and reported he was "electrified." He drove to his dentist, Heinrich Schäfer, with a copy of the article. Dr Schäfer had never heard of sleep apnea but was a born innovator and fabricated a mono-block acrylic device that held the mandible forward, similar to the von Esmarch maneuver[26] (**Fig. 5**). Because side effects of a mandibular advancement appliance (OA$_m$) were unknown, Professor Meier-Ewert wore the original device for 9 months before offering treatment to a patient. By 1984, he had treated 6 patients and presented his findings at the Eighth European Congress on Sleep Research.[27] He introduced the idea of OAT to a European and Asian audience.

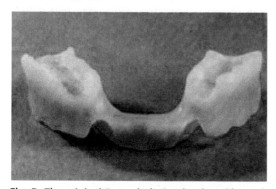

Fig. 5. The original Esmarch device developed by Karlheinz Meier-Ewert, MD, and Heinrich Schäfer, DMD. (*Reprinted by* permission from Springer Nature: Sleep and Breathing. Meier-Ewert Award of the German Society of Dental Sleep Medicine, Susanne Schwarting, ©2006.)

In 1983, Peter George, an orthodontist in Hawaii, attended a meeting with an orthognathic surgeon who found himself in a dilemma because a sleep physician had referred a patient for mandibular advancement surgery to treat severe OSA. The patient had no craniofacial abnormality and the oral surgeon felt that surgery would negatively impact the patient's facial profile and his occlusion. Dr George, well versed in the field of functional orthodontics and appliances used to treat Class II malocclusions, said he could make the patient an appliance that would "keep his jaw forward all night and he [could] take it out in the morning." The first modified activator, later known as the nocturnal airway patency appliance (NAPA) (**Fig. 6**), was placed September 1983 and provided total control of the patient's severe OSA.[28] Peter George and Bruce Soll, the pulmonologist, documented this case in a letter to the *New England Journal of Medicine*[29] published in August of 1985; in it they brought the idea of mandibular advancement OA therapy for OSA to the American medical community.

All of the preceding devices were mono-block, which limited mandibular movement and made alteration of the amount of mandibular advancement difficult. Later in the decade, Howe and McNamara[7–9] changed the face of OAT when they altered the Herbst appliance,[6] making it a removable acrylic device[30] that was also easily adjustable. Now the knowledge and the means were available in the literature, and the way

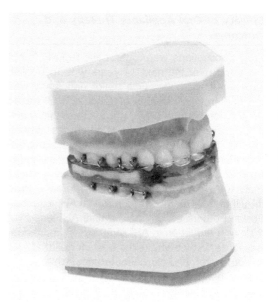

Fig. 6. The NAPA designed by Peter George, DDS. (*Courtesy of* Great Lakes Orthodontics, Tonawanda, NY; with permission.)

was paved for widespread use of OAs in the treatment of OSA.

NEAR HISTORY, 1986 TO 2000: THE ADVENT OF EVIDENCE-BASED DENTISTRY

Before 1986, evidence-based decision making had only a small foothold in dental education. Dentistry had long been taught as an art (ie, copying an instructor's technique), not as a science. Medicine was well ahead of dentistry in this arena, and diagnosis of OSA as a medical disease required dentists to establish themselves on an equal footing with physicians. Into this void came North American researchers, such as Alan Lowe and Glenn Clark; European researchers like Marie Marklund, Joanna Battagel, and Peter R. L'Estrange; and many Japanese dental researchers, including Jiro Kato, Shiro Isono, and Kazuya Yoshida. They undertook analytical evaluation of oral appliances to determine if OAT was a viable treatment for OSA. This pioneering work first looked at efficacy, mechanism of action, anatomic correlates with success of OAT, and adherence to therapy. Many sleep physicians partnered with dentists to analyze the efficacy of individual appliances. By 2000, there were good-quality studies and high enough subject numbers that traditional sleep medicine became more receptive to the use of OAs as an alternative to PAP. The number of designs of Food and Drug Administration (FDA)-cleared OAs increased from a handful to more than 40[31] within 15 years.

Efficacy of Oral Appliance Therapy and Outcomes

Early publications were often case reports,[32] but the trend over the next 14 years was to publish experimental studies. One major deficiency was the numerous definitions of "success" all based on polysomnogram (PSG) parameters; this made it very difficult to compare outcomes among studies. Definitions varied from the classic CPAP definition of a drop in apnea-hypopnea index (AHI) of 50% with a final AHI ≤5 or an AHI less than 10, the surgical definition of merely a drop in AHI greater than 50% with a final AHI less than 20, and others used simply a final AHI less than 20[33] or a reduction in AHI of 50%.[34,35] Evidence-based dentistry became the basis for all that was to come later, and clinical outcomes, while statistically significant, were not always medically significant. Comparative studies between various therapies and OAT were also published.

- OAT versus PAP. The first studies comparing an OA (both prefabricated and custom-fitted)

with PAP in the treatment of mild-moderate OSA were published in 1996 and 1997.[34,35] These studies were prospective and compared not only subjective and objective efficacy, but side effects, compliance, and treatment preference. Although the title stated mild-moderate OSA, the AHI of subjects ranged from 15 to 50, and preference for OAT was strong in those successfully treated with OAT. By 1999, there were 3 crossover treatment trials that showed patients preferred OA over PAP when effectively treated, and adjustable devices were preferred over mono-block devices.[36]
- OAT versus UPPP. Comparison of OA with UPPP outcomes was undertaken by Wilhelmsson and colleagues[37] in 1999; OAT was statistically favored.
- OA versus dissimilar designs. Studies comparing the various groups of devices with each other, that is, TRD versus mandibular repositioning appliances (MRA) [OA$_m$] versus soft-palate lifter, consistently showed that the OA$_m$ was the most effective type of device,[38] and only OA$_m$ produced a consistent improvement in those with severe OSA.[39] Although various designs of OA$_m$ were discussed, regarding the amount of mandibular opening, need for mandibular stabilization, and quantification of mandibular advancement,[40] none of the those empirically tested showed superiority.[41,42]

Mechanism of Action

OA therapy for snoring was initially thought to occur by putting tension on the soft palate to prevent vibration, and researchers were able to show that alteration in airway anatomy allowed adequate treatment of, not only snoring, but OSA.[43,44] Mechanical mandibular advancement was shown to increase airway size and reduce the critical closing pressure (Pcrit) of the passive pharynx in patients during induction of general anesthesia,[45] similar to the technique described by von Esmarch 132 years earlier. Quantifying the amount of mandibular advancement required to open the airway was done first in patients under general anesthesia and was determined to be dose-dependent.[46] Ryan and colleagues[47] measured the cross-sectional area of the upper airway (UA) in awake patients in a supine position while wearing an OA and verified the increase in UA was not predominantly retroglossal, but in the lateral dimension at the level of the velopharynx. This period of research showed us *where* the UA increased in size but did not explain *why* these changes occurred.

Side effects were reported using both questionnaires and dental examination.[48,49] Minor changes in occlusion, altered salivation, discomfort (teeth, muscles, or joint), and occlusal changes increased with the length of OA use. Patients were often unaware of these changes. Pantin and colleagues[48] found that side effects were common but did not appear to lead to discontinuing therapy; of the 14% of patients who had occlusal changes, only half were aware of these alterations. Bondemark[50] concluded that 2 years of treatment had no adverse effects on the craniomandibular status, or temporomandibular joint or function. There was alteration of dental occlusion and slight movement of the mandible. Side effects were thought to be of minor importance but required further, long-term investigation.

Oral Appliance Design

Some of the original studies were done with pre-fabricated devices,[37] others with custom-fitted OAs.[51] Data were gathered more to prove the efficacy of the treatment rather than to analyze the differences among the various OA designs.

Predictors of Success

- Imaging.
  - Screening: Early work looked at using imaging in an attempt to help screen for the presence of OSA by finding a narrow UA or anatomic correlates or to help ascertain the site of obstruction.[52] Controlled studies found gender and positional differences in cephalometric comparisons with control subjects[53]; racial differences were also evident,[40] but findings were often quite heterogeneous. One study found no consistent anatomic difference between those with OSA and a control cohort.[54]
  - Site of obstruction: The site of obstruction was thought to play a role in OAT success[55] because airway size plays a role in airway collapsibility,[56] but it was found not to be a stand-alone predictor of success.[57,58]
  - Correlates with success of OAT: Retrospective studies using cephalometric analysis often identified anatomic differences between those who were successful with OAT and those who failed; both Pcrit and OA successes were found to correlate with the length of the soft palate or hyoid position.[59,60] During this period, imaging was predominantly static 2-dimensional cephalometry. Imaging a dynamic airway that collapses only during sleep with static measures during wakefulness presents

many challenges.[61] Drug-induced sleep endoscopy (DISE) was used early-on to direct surgical intervention,[62] but not applied to OA therapy until the new millennium. Populations in these early studies were small, selection bias was high, and predictive factors were difficult to establish.[43]

- Anthropomorphic and sleep predictors.
  - The influence of anthropomorphic criteria was not consistent from one study to another.[52] Although most patients responded positively to OAT, a significant percentage worsened.[63] Marklund and colleagues[64] identified supine-dependent OSA as a strong predictor of success with OAT.

As we approached the start of the twenty-first century, larger populations were studied and outcomes included both PSG criteria of success as well as quality-of-life (QoL) measures; however, many of these studies were limited by high dropout rates and complete data on only a portion of subjects.[65] Much of the data were not empiric. For example, studies that looked at treating snoring often provided no empiric assessment of snoring,[66] only bed-partner questionnaire responses. Statistical analysis rarely included intent-to-treat, placebo controls, or randomization. But the data were sufficiently adequate that Wolfgang Schmidt-Nowara and colleagues,[67] in their 1995 review, reported that the literature "suggests that oral appliances present a useful alternative, especially for patients with simple snoring and others with moderate OSA who cannot tolerate nasal CPAP." OAs were deemed to be most effective in treating mild-moderate OSA.[68] In his 1999 review, Schmidt-Nowara[36] stated that "it was no longer tenable to label OA therapy an 'experimental' procedure."

MODERN DAY, 2001–2018: MORE AND BETTER RESEARCH...BUT MORE QUESTIONS

As the number of mandibular advancement devices proliferated, so did the science supporting their use in the treatment of OSA. As the design and quality of studies improved, literature reviews became possible. OA therapy was becoming a true medico-dental therapy. Medical advances were driven by the increasing awareness of the epidemic of OSA worldwide, the medical comorbidities, and the determination that appropriate treatment can improve overall health and well-being. OA research over the past 18 years has improved our understanding of the mechanism of action, the side effects, and the improvements in health that relate to OAT.

Medical Advances

Medicine and dentistry have been looking for ways to predict which patients will benefit from a specific therapy for OSA. Although there is a probable genetic basis for OSA, the connection between genes and the observable characteristics of an individual, their phenotype, is impacted by environmental factors, such as stress, disease, and diet, both during embryonic development and throughout life. The search is to identify the specific aspects of an individual's phenotype, for example, symptoms, anatomic correlates, or anthropomorphic findings, that can successfully predict success with OAT.

There are many ways to measure patient phenotypes. Ye and colleagues[69] looked at phenotyping by clinical symptoms and categorized patients as excessively sleepy, minimally symptomatic, or having disturbed sleep. Dentists looked at cephalometric correlates, phenotyping by anatomic findings, for example, a long soft palate, low hyoid bone, or narrowed airway. Presently patients are grouped based on data from a PSG. This includes AHI, oxygen saturation, or level of hypoxia, but the OSA phenotype is much more heterogeneous than differences in AHI.[70] Positional sleep apnea represents a different phenotype from nonpositional OSA,[71] as may rapid eye movement (REM)–dominant OSA.[72] Patients who develop significant hypoxemia with a breathing event are different from those who do not.[73] A low arousal threshold also plays a role in the pathogenesis of OSA.[74] Multiple phenotypes have been identified, but many do not predict OAT outcomes.[75] More recent work by Wellman and his group[76] has tried to combine many of the previous findings into 4 respiratory phenotypes. This work reports that most patients express more than 1 of the 4 respiratory phenotypes, and the proportion of each phenotype expressed varies from person to person. The PALM scale can be determined from data captured during PSG identifying (P)crit, (A)rousal threshold, (L)oop gain, and (M)uscle responsiveness, each of which represents a different etiology of OSA and responds to differing therapies. The PALM scale, coupled with other markers, is expected to aid both physicians and dentists in directing optimal therapy and avoid much of the trial-and-error approach now required to identify patients who will be successful with OAT or other treatments.[77,78] Although none of these prediction methods has yet been validated prospectively, it is one more step toward identifying phenotype classifications that are tied to success with specific therapies.

Outcomes

When PSG parameters were used as the sole outcome criteria for OAT, comparative studies with PAP consistently showed that oral appliances were less effective at improving the oxygen nadir or decreasing the AHI.[79–81] This period saw a slow transition to reporting medical outcomes, relying less on PSG parameters. The 8-year retrospective study of cardiovascular mortality in patients with severe OSA by Anandam and colleagues[82] showed that patients who used an OA had a comparable outcome to those who used PAP. The review by Bratton and colleagues[83] showed that there was no difference between OAs and PAP in improvement in blood pressure. Outcomes in oxidative stress markers and QoL improvements were also seen to be comparable between the 2 treatment options.[84,85] OAT was noninferior to PAP for improvements in mean arterial pressure.[86] QoL outcomes and cognitive testing also showed improvement with OAT,[87] noting no difference in outcome between PAP and OAT.[88,89] OAT therapy was found to be as effective as PAP in controlling symptoms of posttraumatic stress disorder in veterans with OSA.[90] Of note, one study showed a definite inferiority of OA_m to PAP in health outcomes, but used a 1-piece nontitratable OA_m that was not altered by the technician to optimize efficacy.[91] There appears to be no difference in outcomes between PAP and OAT when both therapies are objectively titrated.[92] With the advent of intraoral compliance monitoring, patient reports of hours of use were consistent with self-reported compliance. The average use of an OA was more than 6 to 7 hours per night[63,93–95]; whereas in large international studies, PAP use is closer to 3.3 hours per night.[96,97] This led to the conclusion that higher adherence to OAT, with only partial resolution of PSG parameters, balanced excellent control of disease with PAP used for only a portion of the night.[98,99] Similar findings were found not only in patients with mild-moderate OSA, but also in a significant minority of those with severe OSA.[86]

Long-term positive impacts on PSG findings were pursued. Marklund and colleagues[100] looked at a cohort for more than 5 years and found that, of those initially successful with therapy, the improvement in symptoms and PSG outcomes remained robust at 5 to 10 years. When she looked at more than 15-year follow-up, and controlled for patient weight gain, Marklund[101] found that although the patients remained pleased with treatment and control of snoring, they had almost doubled their baseline AHI in 16 years (from 17 to 32 per hour) and, when the OA was placed, their treated AHI *increased* from 7.2 to 35.1 per hour. Although the number of subjects included was very small, those who used an oral appliance for decades were seen to have a significant exacerbation in their level of OSA. Whether this aggravation of AHI was due to alteration in dental relations such as overjet, or phenotype of the patients, Marklund[101] hypothesized that, similar to CPAP, the amount of mandibular advancement may require continuous titration during long-term treatment.

Titration to Improve Polysomnographic Outcomes

What is found consistently in the literature is that OAs that are titrated for effectiveness[102] outperform those that arbitrarily position the mandible at a single advancement percentage or use maximum comfortable advancement. Positioning the mandible based on symptom relief or the patient's inability to further advance the mandible showed varied responses in AHI decrement. Subjective titration using symptoms is considered less accurate than empiric feedback and many patients report a significant improvement in symptoms without equal improvement in PSG criteria.[103–105]

Studies that titrate OAs objectively, using overnight oximetry at home,[106] sequential home sleep apnea tests,[107–109] a soft pneumatic actuator at home,[110] titration during overnight PSG,[111] or that use hydraulic advancement[112] or metal cables during PSG[88] have found increased improvement beyond results of titration based on symptomatic relief.[113] The outcomes varied widely, and often patient populations were not comparable.

The development of a standardized titration protocol was challenging, because some OAs required removal from the mouth to adjust, whereas others could be adjusted in situ by the technician.[111,113]

Mechanism of Action

Newer studies on the physiology of mandibular advancement gave far more insight into the mechanism of action of OAs. The alteration of UA space appeared to alter both muscle activity[114] and anatomy. The tongue was shown to move forward en bloc in those with a low AHI, following the advanced mandible. However, as the severity of OSA increased, the tongue more often deformed,

resulting in less improvement in UA size. The lateral opening of the UA noted in early scanning studies was postulated to be related to a fibrous attachment from the inner aspect of the mandible to the lateral walls of the UA along, most likely, the pterygomandibular raphé. Alteration in soft tissue position with mandibular advancement appears impacted not only by anatomy and physiology, but also mechanical factors, such as mouth opening.[115] Actual airway size improvement, although variable, was seen at multiple levels.[116,117]

Research on oral appliances focused on mandibular advancement (OA$_m$), and less emphasis was placed on the TRD except in edentulous populations.[b] Comparison studies of OAs with single arch bite plates with no mandibular advancement, favored mandibular protrusion as necessary for significant improvement in sleep parameters.[118,119] During this period, there was renewed investigation into the amount of advancement required for optimal outcomes. The substantial advancement required to open the UA in early studies on anesthetized patients was found not to be universally effective, and some patients required very little advancement for successful treatment with an OA.[109,120,121] Extreme advancement was necessary more often in patients with severe OSA. The precise mechanisms of action are quite complex,[56] and interindividual differences play a significant role. This is an area still poorly understood.[122]

Side Effects

Long-term data were now available. Early studies looked at 1 to 3 years of treatment and found that although the severity of side effects increased with the length of treatment,[123] no difference in side effects was found among various appliance designs; this may vary in widely divergent device designs.[124] Studies looking at 4-year to 15-year data showed an increase in occlusal alteration relative to frequency and length of OA use.[101,125–127] Side effects were noted to be dose-dependent on the amount of mandibular protrusion. Cohen-Levy and colleagues[128] found that forces placed on teeth by mandibular advancement were also dose-dependent and varied between the left and right side. Doff and colleagues[129] found that patients using OAT under the guidance of a qualified dentist actually saw their temporomandibular joint

---

[b]Note: The 2015 American Academy of Sleep Medicine (Ramar) guideline on the use of oral appliances in the treatment of OSA suggests that the consistent term "oral appliance" be used. From this point on, an "oral appliance (OA)," unless specifically noted, will imply a mandibular advancement style of device that is titratable.

function improve. It appeared that most other side effects were short-term or easily controlled. Discontinuing OAT because of perceived side effects was uncommon.[130]

In 2017, the American Academy of Dental Sleep Medicine developed a consensus on the management of side effects created during OAT,[131] classifying side effects into categories of temporomandibular joint–related, intraoral tissue-related, occlusal changes, damage to teeth and restorations, and appliance issues, such as breakage or patient gagging. Their conclusion was that, based on present knowledge, palliative care and watchful waiting were the most reasonable approaches to side-effect management with little need for active intervention.

Oral Appliance Design

Studies of one style of OA versus another became more common; comparison of prefabricated appliances versus custom-fitted appliances, showed clear superiority and patient preference for the fully bespoke device.[132–135] Comparison with non-adjustable mono-block devices showed the superiority of titratable appliances, but the cost of treatment with a titratable device may be higher.[133] It should be noted that many of the mono-block appliances used in studies were altered by a technician, actually rendering them titrated devices, just not titratable by the patient.[136]

Studies that compared one custom-fabricated titratable OA versus a different custom-fabricated OA had diverse outcomes. One study showed a slight statistical difference in early treatment outcomes that became insignificant long-term[137]; others showed no initial statistical difference in outcomes.[138,139] These comparative studies were often difficult to equate because the definitions of success differed from one study to another. Each study had unique criteria for exclusion of subjects and did or did not include subjects with severe OSA.

When a custom-fabricated OA was compared with a placebo device, there was often no difference in daytime sleepiness[140]; this led to an assumption that improvement in daytime sleepiness was, most likely, a placebo effect.[141] Some devices that were more effective in the initial stages of therapy also had higher dropout rates over a 2-year period.[137] One may be more effective in improving PSG parameters, but not be preferred by the patient.[142] Patients appear to prefer appliances that are less bulky and minimize the interincisal vertical opening.[138] Although one might be more effective or more "comfortable" in the first few months, these differences were often lost over time. Comparisons of adjustable versus nonadjustable (mono-block) appliances showed conflicting outcomes in efficacy and adherence. During this period, the American Academy of Dental Sleep Medicine defined an effective oral appliance as one that advances the mandible and allows titration by the patient, because OA_m have been found to be the most effective and widely used in clinical practice.[143]

When Does Individual Design Matter?

Various design elements became an area of research. Does the vertical (interincisal) opening impact efficacy? How far must the mandible be advanced to ensure success? Significant research throughout the past 2 decades showed that increased vertical opening may not necessarily impact treatment success but it does impact patient acceptance,[144] and devices that alter vertical opening without mandibular protrusion may worsen OSA.[141] Further confusing outcome data were the pooling of data from patients using dissimilar appliances.[145,146] Ignoring between-group comparisons could obscure the design features that matter.

- Protrusion: The determination of an arbitrary 75% mandibular advancement required to open the airway in patients under general anesthesia was now shown to overadvance many patients.[109,121] The review by Bartolucci and colleagues[120] of 13 randomized controlled studies looking at effective advancement, showed no statistical difference in outcomes when the mandible was advanced more than 50%. Because many studies start titration at an advanced position of 75%, it is possible that dentists limit successful outcomes by overadvancing many patients with less severe OSA.
- Vertical opening: In studies that use the same custom-made OA in both experimental arms with alteration of design features was first done in 1998.[147] Because this study altered both the amount of mandibular protrusion and the vertical opening, it was not possible to determine exactly why more patients had a more positive outcome at 70% advancement than at 100% advancement. To date, no study has evaluated the vertical opening of an OA in relation to the mandibular angle of the patient, but there is concern that a steep mandibular angle may actually lead to aggravation of OSA with vertical opening.[122,148]
- Stabilization of the mandible: Norrhem and Marklund[149] added elastics to an appliance to limit mouth opening and found improved outcomes in those with severe OSA. Milano and colleagues[150] also added elastics to a single OA design and almost doubled the

percentage of patients effectively treated. One crossover study compared 2 different devices at the same protrusion and same vertical opening; despite no cephalometric differences, the mono-block was found to be more effective in reducing AHI than was the twin-block, which did not prevent mouth opening (final AHI 5.9 vs 15.2).[151] Maintaining mandibular closure appears to be an important design feature in OAT when compared to an appliance that allows mandibular opening.[149,152]

The style of mechanics for advancement (propulsion vs traction) does not seem to alter outcomes. Design does not appear to impact the *severity* of side effects.[153] Experimental studies that show differences in outcomes and attempt to control for subject variability, as well as studies comparing one style of device with another, indicate that OA design features do matter, but the exact features that are responsible are elusive.[137,139,142]

Predictors of Success

To determine who will be effectively treated with OAT is important. Because as many as 50% of subjects discontinue use of an OA in the first year,[154] proper allocation of medical resources requires a better understanding of what prognostic factors exist for OAT success.

- Imaging
  - Cephalometric correlates have been sought for more than 30 years, and the results have been very heterogeneous. Some studies have found that mandibular plane angle, length of soft palate,[155,156] position of hyoid bone, or any of a multiple of measurements were correlated with OA success. However, these were not predictive of OA efficacy when controlling for anthropomorphic measurements, such as body mass index,[157] sex,[158] age,[159] or neck circumference.[118] Anthropomorphic and physiologic predictors have limited clinical utility in predicting OA success,[103,160] as has baseline AHI.[146] Although reviews have shown that many findings were associated with the *presence* of OSA (UA size, lower hyoid position,[161] or a long lower face), these studies did not help to influence the choice of therapy.[162]
  - Three-dimensional imaging: Scanning of patients with MRI during the Mueller maneuver, with and without mandibular advancement,[163] was hoped to predict OA efficacy. What 3-dimensional scanning has allowed is the development of computer-aided design models that allow mathematical evaluation of the airway. Computational fluid dynamics (CFD) has been used to determine the alteration in airflow velocity with and without mandibular advancement.[122] Correlation between predicted outcomes with CFD and actual outcomes with OAT have shown this technique to be a potential tool for prediction of OA success.[164,165]
  - Dynamic imaging: Videoendoscopy showed that the limiting factor in OA success appeared to be retropalatal changes and that awake patients with circumferential retropalatal collapse of the UA have a high probability of failing OAT.[166] Oropharyngeal collapse without velopharyngeal collapse appeared to correlate with OAT success,[167] but predictive criteria have not been determined.
  - DISE has been used visualize the airway changes that occur with mandibular advancement. This technique is subjective, requires pharmaceutical agents that impact airway function,[168] and is invasive, which limits its use.
  - The location of the narrowest part of the pharyngeal airway with acoustic pharyngometry was also found not to be predictive of OA success.[169]
- Clinical features: Various clinical features also have been linked to OAT failure, including a high mean diastolic blood pressure and low sleep-time oxygen nadir.[170] Although one study found that nasal abnormalities negatively impact OA success,[159] others have shown no PSG, demographic, anthropomorphic, cephalometric, or otorhinolaryngological parameters that reliably predicted OA success.[171]
- CPAP pressures predict UA collapsibility,[172] therefore the level of CPAP pressure has also been considered as a possible predictor of OA success. Higher required CPAP pressures have been found to correlate with a decreased effectiveness of OAT. There appears to be a significant racial difference between an Asian and a primarily White cohort in required PAP pressures. Others found only a weak dependence on the severity of the OSA and effective PAP pressures.[173–176]
- Newer research shows that the inspiratory airflow shape recorded during PSG is influenced by pharyngeal structure and helps to identify the site of obstruction during natural sleep in various sleep positions.[177] Information from routine PSG may eventually help predict the efficacy of OAT.
- Pretreatment mechanical overnight titration: Automated titration, before fabrication of an

OA is also hoped to predict who will be successful with mandibular advancement and aid identification of the effective mandibular position. Kuna and colleagues[178] found that their titration device identified patients who would be successful with OAT, but fewer than half of their subjects were actually treated effectively. Use of a step motor showed moderate sensitivity but high specificity when identifying patients who would be appropriately treated,[179] but does not necessarily identify the ideal mandibular position.[160] Mechanical titration techniques are often highly technique sensitive. They do not allow the use of the patient's own custom-fabricated OA, often prevent mouth closure, and normally require overnight laboratory testing.

The site of obstruction varies with patient position,[64,146,180,181] and airway dynamics change with sleep onset. We still are unable to predict who will be successful with OAT. Many of these potential prediction methods have given inconsistent outcomes or are not clinically accessible to all practitioners.[182]

Predictors of Adherence

As with PAP,[183] adherence to therapy is a significant problem. OA adherence is highest in thinner, younger[184] subjects with few or no nasal obstructions.[159] One study could verify that only 26% of patients continued to use the OA after 7 years,[185] whereas another reported that only 37% of the subjects continued to use the OA nightly.[186] Others showed even higher adherence, with 57.7% of patients with severe sleep apnea using the OA long-term.[187] Some mono-block appliances have very poor adherence, with only 50% of subjects using the device even part time at 7 months after placement and only 12% still using the OA at 12 months.[154] OA adherence is higher with adjustable devices that allow some mandibular movement.[95,145] One study found adherence correlated with the length of the mandible.[188] Zarhin and Oksenberg[189] showed that PAP adherence is contingent on diverse factors, including emotional discomfort and expectation of a cure rather than self-management. Johal and colleagues[135] stressed that OA therapy is entirely patient-dependent, and an overriding principle in its success must be patient comfort and consequent use. Dieltjens and colleagues[190] assessed patients with a type D personality and found they were 3 times more likely to discontinue OAT than patients without a type D personality. PAP compliance has been found to be higher in a sleep center setting than in a primary care setting.[191] This may also be true of treatment from a qualified dentist rather than a dentist unaware of the impact of OSA. We do not know if patients are more adherent to therapy when treated by a dentist well versed in the area of DSM. We do know that short-term control of OSA by OA was predictive of long-term (1000 days) efficiency[145] and, although adherence to OAT appears related mostly to improvement in symptoms,[154] efforts to predict OA adherence have, so far, been unsuccessful.[192]

New OAs as well as novel tongue retainers have poured on to the market.[193] Over the past 2 decades, the list of FDA-cleared devices grew from fewer than 40 to more than 150.[194]

Better-designed studies with larger populations, and placebo-controlled using objective compliance monitoring are now the norm. Less heterogeneous outcome definitions allowed systematic reviews. The overall quality of the literature has improved. In 2006, Ferguson[81] summarized a literature review with, "published literature now provides evidence for the efficacy of OAs in the treatment of patients with mild to moderate OSA. They play a role in a selected group of patients in whom an alternative to CPAP is desired."

Given the present level of technology, OAs appear to have medical outcomes comparable with PAP. Custom-fitted appliances empirically titrated for efficacy provide optimal results. Adherence is high in those who are adequately treated, but there is, as of yet, no easy, inexpensive effective way to predict who will be adequately treated and who will continue to use an OA long-term.

Patient-centered measures are playing a greater role in studies about OAs. Early studies were done to ascertain the efficacy of therapy and recent studies show comparable outcomes to established therapies. Now the studies must involve patients in decisions about therapeutic choice,[135] as well as improving the identification of patients more likely to be effectively treated and adherent to long-term care.

QUESTIONS FOR THE FUTURE
Medical Advances

Biomarkers

Much effort has gone into identifying biologic markers that are indicative of OSA.[195] These surrogate markers, once identified, could be used to screen large populations for OSA before final diagnosis using overnight testing or as a proxy for overnight testing. Unfortunately, no individual biomarkers have performed sufficiently well to warrant clinical implementation. Current research efforts into OSA prediction focus on using bioinformatics approaches to identify multi-biomarker footprints, genetic expression that may allow identification of individuals at risk for developing complications from OSA or assess their outcomes of treatment.[196] For example, researchers have started to look at microRNA profiles as an indicator of CPAP response.[197] Could there be similar markers for response to OAT? This could help contain costs, ease delays in diagnosis, and personalize treatment.

Determine who requires treatment

As the number of people who are diagnosed with OSA increases, the medical field attempts to determine if all patients require treatment. Studies have shown that patients who are not sleepy may not receive any health improvement from intervention.[198] Is sleepiness a critical part of the problem? Do medical outcomes improve with every therapy?[199] Does combining various therapies improve outcomes? Are there patients who will not benefit from present therapies for OSA, and development of new therapies will provide improved outcomes?

Phenotyping

Can personalized phenotyping account for all previous findings of OA success based on respiratory parameters, subtypes of positional OSA, gender, age, anthropomorphic data, imaging data, race, hormone status, and parse out which patient will be adequately treated with OAT? Future therapeutic decisions are no longer expected to base treatment options only on AHI, symptoms severity, and comorbidities.[61,200] A phenotypic model has the potential to shift the current CPAP-as-first-line-treatment approach to non-PAP alternatives for a substantial proportion of appropriately selected patients with OSA.[61,201]

Because a patient's personality, expectations, and support system all play a role in adherence to therapy, can it be determined who is most likely to use an OA long-term, making the treatment cost-effective?

The field requires unified, consistent definitions of success for the treatment of OSA, definitions that can be applied to all therapeutic approaches. Although we may always use PSG parameters, finding biomarkers that require less expensive or intensive testing would be ideal.

Device Design

Can phenotyping incorporate anatomy and personality factors to determine which design of OA would be most effective for individual patients? Can research determine how appliance design features impact patient anatomy or adherence to therapy?

Can we develop new, less labor-intensive, testing that will accurately determine the ideal mandibular advancement and interincisal distance required by each patient?

Just as the past 150 years have laid the groundwork for where the field of DSM is at present, the future will continue to be an amalgam of popular cultural beliefs and increasing patient awareness of the need for treatment as the medical burden of OSA continues to escalate. Sleep medicine will continue to advance with establishment of standardized definitions of success and new and better ways to screen for, diagnose, and treat OSA. Dentistry, based on the latest medical and dental knowledge, will continue to screen for the presence of OSA and provide ever more effective and targeted therapy. Continued research in OA design will provide optimal care for each appropriate patient.

ACKNOWLEDGMENTS

The author expresses her appreciation to Alice C. Grover, Kelly Carden, MD, Karlheinz Meier-Ewert, MD, Susanne Schwarting, DMD and Peter George, DDS for their assistance with this article.

REFERENCES

1. Catlin G. Breath of Life {All life (on earth) is breath and all else (on earth) is death}. (Manugraph). London: Tribner & Co; 1861. p. 15–30 (Available on Google Books).
2. Clover JT. Chloroform accidents. Br Med J 1871; 2(549):33–4.
3. Esmarch V. Handbuch der Kriegschirurgischen Technik. Eine gekrönte Preisschrift. Hannover (Germany): Carl Rŭmpler; 1877. p. 112–25 (Available on Google Books).
4. Defalque RJ, Wright AJ. Who invented the "jaw thrust"? Anesthesiology 2003;99(6):1463–4.
5. Robin P. La chute de la base de la langue consideree comme une nouvelle cause de gene dans la respiration naso-pharyngienne. Bull Acad Med 1923;89:37–41 (Translation by Alice C. Grover 2014).
6. Pancherz H. History, background and development of the Herbst appliance. Semin Orthod 2003;9(1):3–11.
7. McNamara JA, Howe RP. Clinical management of the acrylic splint Herbst appliance. Am J Orthod Dentofac Orthop 1988;94:142–9.
8. Howe RP, McNamara JA. Clinical management of the Herbst appliance. J Clin Orthod 1983;17:456–63.
9. Howe RP. Updating the bonded Herbst appliance. J Clin Orthod 1983;17:122–4.

10. Schossow GW. Patent application with USPTO- anti snoring device. 1984. Available at: http://patft.uspto.gov/netacgi/nph-Parser?Sect1=PTO1&Sect2=HITOFF&d=PALL&p=1&u=%2Fnetahtml%2FPTO%2Fsrchnum.htm&r=1&f=G&l=50&s1=4551473.PN.&OS=PN/4551473&RS=PN/4551473. Accessed December 9, 2017.

11. Shaw LH. Application for patent USPTO- anti-snoring chin spring 1891. Available at: http://pdfpiw.uspto.gov/.piw?Docid=00460451&homeurl=http%3A%2F%2Fpatft.uspto.gov%2Fnetacgi%2Fnph-Parser%3FSect1%3DPTO1%2526Sect2%3DHITOFF%2526d%3DPALL%2526p%3D1%2526u%3D%25252Fnetahtml%25252FPTO%25252Fsrchnum.htm%2526r%3D1%2526f%3DG%2526l%3D50%2526s1%3D0460451.PN.%2526OS%3DPN%2F0460451%2526RS%3DPN%2F0460451&PageNum=&Rtype=&SectionNum=&idkey=NONE&Input=View+first+page. Accessed December 9, 2017.

12. Wilson GH. Application for US Patent – nasal dilator. 1918. Available at: http://pdfpiw.uspto.gov/.piw?Docid=01256188&homeurl=http%3A%2F%2Fpatft.uspto.gov%2Fnetacgi%2Fnph-Parser%3FSect1%3DPTO1%2526Sect2%3DHITOFF%2526d%3DPALL%2526p%3D1%2526u%3D%25252Fnetahtml%25252FPTO%25252Fsrchnum.htm%2526r%3D1%2526f%3DG%2526l%3D50%2526s1%3D1256188.PN.%2526OS%3DPN%2F1256188%2526RS%3DPN%2F1256188&PageNum=&Rtype=&SectionNum=&idkey=NONE&Input=View+first+page. Accessed December 12, 2017.

13. Moulton SA. US patent application for lip shield 1903. Available at: http://pdfpiw.uspto.gov/.piw?Docid=00746869&homeurl=http%3A%2F%2Fpatft.uspto.gov%2Fnetacgi%2Fnph-Parser%3FSect1%3DPTO1%2526Sect2%3DHITOFF%2526d%3DPALL%2526p%3D1%2526u%3D%25252Fnetahtml%25252FPTO%25252Fsrchnum.htm%2526r%3D1%2526f%3DG%2526l%3D50%2526s1%3D0746869.PN.%2526OS%3DPN%2F0746869%2526RS%3DPN%2F0746869&PageNum=&Rtype=&SectionNum=&idkey=NONE&Input=View+first+page. Accessed December 10, 2017.

14. Anderson S. US patent Application for anti-snoring mouthpiece. 1897. Available at: http://pdfpiw.uspto.gov/.piw?PageNum=0&docid=00587358&IDKey=6C482210C27A%0D%0A&HomeUrl=http%3A%2F%2Fpatft.uspto.gov%2Fnetacgi%2Fnph-Parser%3FSect1%3DPTO1%2526Sect2%3DHITOFF%2526d%3DPALL%2526p%3D1%2526u%3D%25252Fnetahtml%25252FPTO%25252Fsrchnum.htm%2526r%3D1%2526f%3DG%2526l%3D50%2526s1%3D0587358.PN.%2526OS%3DPN%2F0587358%2526RS%3DPN%2F0587358. Accessed December 1, 2017.

15. King EG. US patent application for oral 'respirator.' 1927. Available at: http://pdfpiw.uspto.gov/.piw?Docid=01674336&homeurl=http%3A%2F%2Fpatft.uspto.gov%2Fnetacgi%2Fnph-Parser%3FSect1%3DPTO1%2526Sect2%3DHITOFF%2526d%3DPALL%2526p%3D1%2526u%3D%25252Fnetahtml%25252FPTO%25252Fsrchnum.htm%2526r%3D1%2526f%3DG%2526l%3D50%2526s1%3D1674336.PN.%2526OS%3DPN%2F1674336%2526RS%3DPN%2F1674336&PageNum=&Rtype=&SectionNum=&idkey=NONE&Input=View+first+page. Accessed December 12, 2017.

16. Corniello G. US patent application for soft palate lifter. 1962. Available at: http://pdfpiw.uspto.gov/.piw?PageNum=0&docid=03132647&IDKey=C0A38CF3E455%0D%0A&HomeUrl=http%3A%2F%2Fpatft.uspto.gov%2Fnetacgi%2Fnph-Parser%3FSect1%3DPTO1%2526Sect2%3DHITOFF%2526d%3DPALL%2526p%3D1%2526u%3D%25252Fnetahtml%25252FPTO%25252Fsrchnum.htm%2526r%3D1%2526f%3DG%2526l%3D50%2526s1%3D3132647.PN.%2526OS%3DPN%2F3132647%2526RS%3DPN%2F3132647. Accessed December 10, 2017.

17. Lavie P. Who was the first to use the term Pickwickian in connection with sleepy patients? History of sleep apnoea syndrome. Sleep Med Rev 2008; 12:5–17.

18. Dickens C. The posthumous papers of the Pickwick Club. London: Chapman and Hall; 1837.

19. Kuhl W. History of clinical research on the sleep apnea syndrome. Respiration 1997;64(suppl I):5–10.

20. Guilleminault CA, Eldridge FL, Dement WC. Insomnia with sleep apnea: a new syndrome. Science 1973;181:856–8.

21. Remmers JE, DeGroot WJ, Sauerland EK, et al. Pathogenesis of upper airway occlusion during sleep. J Appl Physiol Respir Environ Exerc Physiol 1978;44(6):931–8.

22. Walsh RE, Michaelson ED, Harkleroad LE, et al. Upper airway obstruction in obese patients with sleep disturbance and somnolence. Ann Int Med 1972;76:185–92.

23. Sullivan C, Berthon-Jones M, Issa F, et al. Reversal of obstructive sleep apnoea by continuous positive airway pressure applied through the nares. Lancet 1981;317(8225):862–5.

24. Samelson C. US Patent office application for Tongue retaining device. 1979. Available at: http://patft.uspto.gov/netacgi/nph-Parser?Sect1=PTO1&Sect2=HITOFF&d=PALL&p=1&u=%2Fnetahtml%2FPTO%2Fsrchnum.htm&r=1&f=G&l=50&s1=4169473.PN.&OS=PN/4169473&RS=PN/4169473.

25. Cartwright RD, Samelson CF. The effects of a nonsurgical treatment for obstructive sleep apnea. The tongue retaining device. JAMA 1982;248:705–70.

26. Schwarting S. Meier-Ewert award of the German Society of Dental Sleep Medicine. Sleep Breath 2006;10:57–61.

27. Meier-Ewert K, Schäfer WK, Kloss W [abstract]. Treatment of sleep apnea by a mandibular protracting device, 217. München (Germany): 7th Europ Sleep Res Soc Congress; 1984.

28. George PT. Lifetime achievement award acceptance speech (or the genesis of the AADSM). Dialogue 2006;2:19–20.

29. Soll BA, George PT. Treatment of obstructive sleep apnea with a nocturnal apnea patency appliance. N Engl J Med 1985;313(6):386.

30. Howe RP. Removable plastic Herbst retainer. J Clin Orthod 1987;21(8):533–7.

31. FDA Premarket notification. Available at: https://www.accessdata.fda.gov/scripts/cdrh/cfdocs/cfPMN/pmn.cfm.

32. Clark GT, Arand D, Chung E, et al. Effect of mandibular positioning on obstructive sleep apnea. Am Rev Respir Dis 1993;147(3):624–9.

33. O'Sullivan RA, Hillman DR, Mateljan R, et al. Mandibular advancement splint: an appliance to treat snoring and obstructive sleep apnea. Am J Respir Crit Care Med 1995;151:194–8.

34. Ferguson KA, Ono T, Lowe AA, et al. A short-term controlled trial of an adjustable oral appliance for the treatment of mild to moderate obstructive sleep apnea. Thorax 1997;52(4):362–8.

35. Ferguson KA, Ono T, Lowe AA, et al. A randomized crossover study of an oral appliance vs nasal-continuous positive airway pressure in the treatment of mild-moderate obstructive sleep apnea. Chest 1996;109(5):1269–75.

36. Schmidt-Nowara WW. Recent developments in oral appliance therapy of sleep disordered breathing. Sleep Breath 1999;3(3):103–6.

37. Wilhelmsson B, Tegelberg Å, Walker-Engström ML, et al. A prospective randomized study of a dental appliance compared with uvulopalatopharyngoplasty in the treatment of obstructive sleep apnea. Acta Otolaryngol 1999;119(4):503–9.

38. Hans MG, Nelson S, Luks VG, et al. Comparison of two dental devices for treatment for obstructive sleep apnea syndrome (OSAS). Am J Orthod Dentofacial Orthop 1997;111(5):562–70.

39. Barthlen GM, Brown LK, Wiland MR, et al. Comparison of three oral appliances for treatment of severe obstructive sleep apnea. Sleep Med 2000;1(4):299–305.

40. Liu Y, Park Y-C, Lowe AA, et al. Supine cephalometric analyses of an adjustable oral appliances used in the treatment of obstructive sleep apnea. Sleep Breath 2000;4(2):59–66.

41. Eckhart J. Comparisons of oral devices for snoring. J Calif Dent Assoc 1998;26:611–23.

42. Menn SJ, Loube DI, Morgan TD, et al. The mandibular repositioning device: role in the treatment of obstructive sleep apnea. Sleep 1996;19(10):794–800.

43. Lévy P, Pépin JL, Mayer P, et al. Management of simple snoring, upper airway resistance syndrome and moderate sleep apnea syndrome. Sleep 1996;19(9):S101–10.

44. Bonham PE, Currier GF, Orr WC, et al. The effect of a modified functional appliance on obstructive sleep apnea. Am J Orthod Dentofac Orthop 1988;94:384–92.

45. Isono S, Tanaka A, Sho Y, et al. Advancement of the mandible improves velopharyngeal airway patency. J Appl Physiol (1985) 1995;79(6):2132–8.

46. Kato J, Isono S, Tanaka A, et al. Dose-dependent effects of mandibular advancement on pharyngeal mechanics and nocturnal oxygenation in patients with sleep-disordered breathing. Chest 2000;17:1065–72.

47. Ryan CF, Love LL, Fleetham JA, et al. Mandibular advancement oral appliance therapy for obstructive sleep apnoea: effect on awake caliber of the velopharynx. Thorax 1999;54(11):972–7.

48. Pantin CC, Hillman DR, Tennant M. Dental side effects of an oral device to treat snoring and obstructive sleep apnea. Sleep 1999;22(2):237–40.

49. Shadaba A, Battagel JM, Owa A, et al. Evaluation of the Herbst advancement splint in the management of patients with sleep-related breathing disorders. Clin Otolaryngol 2000;25(5):404–12.

50. Bondemark L. Does 2 years' nocturnal treatment with a mandibular advancement splint in adult patients with snoring and OSAS cause a change in the posture of the mandible? Am J Orthod Dentofacial Orthop 1999;116:621–8.

51. Clark GT, Blumenfeld I, Yaffe N, et al. A crossover study comparing the efficacy of continuous positive airway pressure with anterior mandibular positioning devices on patients with obstructive sleep apnea. Chest 1996;109(6):1477–83.

52. Lowe AA, Ono T, Ferguson KA, et al. Cephalometric comparisons of craniofacial and upper airway structure by skeletal subtype and gender in patients with obstructive sleep apnea. Am J Orthod Dentofacial Orthop 1996;110(6):653–64.

53. Lowe AA, Özbek MM, Miyamoto K, et al. Cephalometric and demographic characteristics of obstructive sleep apnea: an evaluation with partial least squares analysis. Angle Orthod 1997;67(2):143–54.

54. Mayer G, Meier-Ewert K. Cephalometric predictors for orthopedic mandibular advancement in obstructive sleep apnea. Eur J Orthod 1995;17(1):35–43.

55. Ishida M, Inoue Y, Suto Y, et al. Mechanism of action and therapeutic indication of prosthetic mandibular advancement in obstructive sleep apnea syndrome. Psychiatry Clin Neurosci 1998;52(2):227–9.

56. De Backer JW, Vos WG, Verhulst AL, et al. Novel imaging techniques using computer methods for the evaluation of the upper airway in patients with

sleep disordered breathing: a comprehensive review. Sleep Med Rev 2008;12(6):437–47.

57. Henke KG, Frantz DE, Kuna ST. An oral elastic mandibular advancement device for obstructive sleep apnea. Am J Respir Crit Care Med 2000; 161:420–5.

58. Liu Y, Lowe A, Fleetham JA, et al. Cephalometric and physiologic predictors of the efficacy of an adjustable oral appliance for treating obstructive sleep apnea. Am J Orthod Dentofacial Orthop 2001;120(6):639–47.

59. Sforza E, Bacon W, Weiss T, et al. Upper airway collapsibility and cephalometric variables in patients with obstructive sleep apnea. Am J Respir Crit Care Med 2000;161:347–52.

60. Eveloff SE, Rosenberg CL, Carlisle CE, et al. Efficacy of a Herbst mandibular advancement device in obstructive sleep apnea. Am J Respir Crit Care Med 1994;149(4):905–9.

61. Eckert DJ. Phenotypic approaches to obstructive sleep apnoea—new pathways for targeted therapy. Sleep Med Rev 2018;37:45–59.

62. Pringle MB, Croft CB. A grading system for patients with obstructive sleep apnea—based on sleep nasendoscopy. Clin Otolaryngol 1993;18(6):480–4.

63. Lowe AA, Sjöholm TT, Ryan CF, et al. Treatment, airway and compliance effects of a titratable oral appliance. Sleep 2000;23(Suppl 4):S172–8.

64. Marklund M, Persson M, Franklin KA. Treatment success with a mandibular advancement device is related to supine dependent sleep apnea. Chest 1998;114:1630–5.

65. Pancer J, Al-faifi A, Al-Faifi M, et al. Evaluation of variable mandibular advancement appliance for treatment of snoring and sleep apnea. Chest 1999;116:1511–8.

66. Deary V, Ellis JG, Wilson JA, et al. Simple snoring: not quite so simple after all? Sleep Med Rev 2014; 18(6):453–62.

67. Schmidt-Nowara WW, Lowe AA, Wiegand L, et al. Oral appliances for the treatment of snoring and obstructive sleep apnea: a review. Sleep 1995; 18(6):501–10.

68. Schmidt-Nowara WW, Meade TE, Hayes MB. Treatment of snoring and obstructive sleep apnea with dental orthosis. Chest 1991;99(6):1378–85.

69. Ye L, Pien GW, Ratcliffe SJ, et al. The different clinical faces of obstructive sleep apnoea: a cluster analysis. Eur Respir J 2014;44:1600–7.

70. Bianchi MT, Russo K, Gabbidon H, et al. Big data in sleep medicine: prospects and pitfalls in phenotyping. Nat Sci Sleep 2017;9:11–29.

71. Oksenberg A. Positional patients (PP) and non-positional patients (NPP) are two dominant phenotypes that should be included in the phenotypic approaches to obstructive sleep apnea. Sleep Med Rev 2018;37:173–4.

72. Mokhleski B, Punjabi NM. "REM-related" obstructive sleep apnea: an epiphenomenon or a clinically important entity? Sleep 2012;35(1):5–7.

73. Palma JA, Iriarte J, Fernandez S, et al. Characterizing the phenotypes of obstructive sleep apnea: clinical, sleep, and autonomic features of obstructive sleep apnea with and without hypoxia. Clin Neurophysiol 2014;125:1783–91.

74. Younes M. Role of respiratory control mechanisms in the pathogenesis of obstructive sleep apnea. J Appl Physiol (1985) 2008;105(5):1389–405.

75. Sutherland K, Takaya H, Qian J, et al. Oral appliance treatment response and polysomnographic phenotypes of obstructive sleep apnea. J Clin Sleep Med 2015;11(8):861–868G.

76. Wellman A, Edwards BA, Sands SA, et al. A simplified method for determining phenotypic traits in patients with obstructive sleep apnea. J Appl Physiol 2013;114(7):911–22.

77. Carberry JC, Amartoury J, Eckert D. Personalized management approach for OSA. Chest 2018; 153(3):744–55.

78. Eckert D, White DP, Jordan AS, et al. Defining phenotypic caused of obstructive sleep apnea. Am J Respir Crit Care Med 2013;188(8):996–1004.

79. Hoekema A, Stagenga A, de Bont LGM. Efficacy and co-morbidity of oral appliances in the treatment of obstructive sleep apnea-hypopnea: a systematic review. Crit Rev Oral Biol Med 2005;15(3):137–55.

80. Hoekema A, Stegenga B, Wijkstra PJ, et al. Obstructive sleep apnea therapy. J Dent Res 2008;87(9):882–7.

81. Ferguson KA, Cartwright R, Rogers R, et al. Oral appliances for snoring and obstructive sleep apnea: a review. Sleep 2006;29(2):244–62.

82. Anandam A, Patil A, Akinnusi M, et al. Cardiovascular mortality in obstructive sleep apnea treated with continuous positive airway pressure or oral appliance: an observational study. Respiration 2013;18(8):1184–90.

83. Bratton DJ, Gaisel T, Wons AM, et al. CPAP vs mandibular advancement devices and blood pressure in patients with obstructive sleep apnea. A systemic review and meta-analysis. JAMA 2015; 314(21):2280–93.

84. Dal-Fabbro C, Garbuio S, D'Almeida V, et al. Mandibular advancement device and CPAP upon cardiovascular parameters in OSA. Sleep Breath 2012;18(4):749–59.

85. Hoekema A, Voors AA, Wijkstra PJ, et al. Effects of oral appliances and CPAP on the left ventricle and natriuretic peptides. Int J Cardiol 2008;128(2):232–9.

86. Phillips CL, Grunstein RR, Darendeliler MA, et al. Health outcomes of continuous positive airway pressure versus oral appliance treatment for obstructive sleep apnea; a randomized controlled trial. Am J Respir Crit Care Med 2013;187(8):879–87.

87. Johal A. Health-related quality of life in patients with sleep-disordered breathing: effect of mandibular advancement appliances. J Prosthet Dent 2006; 96(4):298–302.

88. Gagnadoux F, Fleury B, Vielle B, et al. Titrated mandibular advancement versus positive airway pressure for sleep apnoea. Eur Respir J 2009; 34(4):914–20.

89. Doff M, Hoekema A, Wijkstra PJ, et al. Oral appliance versus continuous positive airway pressure in obstructive sleep apnea syndrome: a 2-year follow-up. Sleep 2013;36(9):1289–96.

90. El-Solh AA, Hornish GG, Ditursi G, et al. A randomized crossover trial evaluating continuous positive airway pressure versus mandibular advancement device on health outcomes in veterans with posttraumatic stress disorder. J Clin Sleep Med 2017;13(11):1327–35.

91. Lam B, Sam K, Mok WYK, et al. Randomized study of three non-surgical treatments in mild to moderate obstructive sleep apnea. Thorax 2007;62(4):354–9.

92. Aarab G, Lobbezoo F, Hamburger HL, et al. Oral appliance therapy versus nasal continuous positive airway pressure in obstructive sleep apnea: a randomized, placebo-controlled trial. Respiration 2011;81(5):411–9.

93. Vanderveken OM, Dieltjens M, Wouters K, et al. Objective measurement of compliance during oral appliance therapy for sleep-disordered breathing. Thorax 2013;68(1):91–6.

94. Dieltjens M, Verbruggen AE, Braem MJ, et al. Determinants of objective compliance during oral appliance therapy in patients with sleep-disordered breathing–a prospective clinical trial. JAMA Otolaryngol Head Neck Surg 2015;14(10):894–900.

95. Bachour P, Bachour A, Kauppi P, et al. Oral appliance in sleep apnea treatment: respiratory and clinical effects and long-term adherence. Sleep Breath 2016;20:805–12.

96. McEvoy RD, Antic NA, Heeley E, et al. CPAP for prevention of cardiovascular events in obstructive sleep apnea. N Engl J Med 2016;375(10):919–31.

97. Mokhlesi B, Ayas NT. Cardiovascular events in obstructive sleep apnea—can CPAP therapy SAVE lives? N Engl J Med 2016;375(10):994–6.

98. Sutherland K, Phillips C, Cistulli PA. Efficacy versus effectiveness in the treatment of obstructive sleep apnea. J Dent Sleep Med 2015;2(4):175–81.

99. Edwards BA, Wellman A, Owens RL. PSGs: more than AHI. J Clin Sleep Med 2013;9(6):527–8.

100. Marklund M, Sahlin C, Stenlund H, et al. Mandibular advancement, device in patients with obstructive sleep apnea. Long-term effects on apnea and asleep. Chest 2001;120(1):162–9.

101. Marklund M. Long-term efficacy of an oral appliance in early treated patients with obstructive sleep apnea. Sleep Breath 2016;20(2):689–94.

102. Aarab G, Nikolopoulou M, Ahlberg J, et al. Oral appliance therapy versus nasal continuous positive airway pressure in obstructive sleep apnea: a randomized, placebo-controlled trial on psychological distress. Clin Oral Investig 2017;21(7):2371–8.

103. Campbell AJ, Reynolds G, Tengrove H, et al. Mandibular advancement splint titration in obstructive sleep apnea. Sleep Breath 2009;13:157–62.

104. Engleman HM, McDonald JP, Graham D, et al. Randomized crossover trial of two treatments for sleep apnea/hypopnea syndrome. Am J Respir Crit Care Med 2002;166:855–9.

105. Neill A, Whyman R, Bannan S, et al. Mandibular splint improves indices of obstructive sleep apnoea and snoring but side effects are common. N Z Med J 2002;115(1156):1–8.

106. Fleury B, Rakotonanhary D, Pételle B, et al. Mandibular advancement titration for obstructive sleep apnea: optimization of the procedure by combining clinical and oximetric parameters. Chest 2004;125:1761–7.

107. Levendowski DJ, Morgan TD, Patrickus JE, et al. In-home evaluation of efficacy and titration of a mandibular advancement device for obstructive sleep apnea. Sleep Breath 2007;11:139–47.

108. Gindre L, Gagnadoux F, Meslier N, et al. Mandibular advancement for obstructive sleep apnea: dose effect on apnea, long-term use and tolerance. Respiration 2008;76(4):386–92.

109. AARAB G, Lobbezoo F, Hamburger HL, et al. Effects of an oral appliance with different mandibular protrusion positions at a constant vertical dimension on obstructive sleep apnea. Clin Oral Investig 2010;14(3):339–45.

110. Brugarolis R, Valero-Sarmiento JM, Bozhurt A, et al. Auto-adjusting mandibular repositioning device for in-home use. Conf Proc IEEE Eng Med Biol Soc 2016;4296–9. https://doi.org/10.1109/EMBC.2016.7591677.

111. Holley AB, Lettieri CJ, Shah AA. Efficacy of an adjustable oral appliance and comparison to continuous positive airway pressure for the treatment of obstructive sleep apnea syndrome. Chest 2011;140(6):1511–6.

112. Pételle B, Vincent G, Gagnadoux F, et al. One-night mandibular advancement titration for obstructive sleep apnea syndrome. Am J Respir Crit Care Med 2002;165:1150–3.

113. Almeida FR, Parker JA, Hodges JS, et al. Effect of titration polysomnogram on treatment success with a mandibular repositioning appliance. J Clin Sleep Med 2009;5(3):198–204.

114. Johal A, Gill G, Ferman A, et al. The effect of mandibular advancement appliances on awake upper airway and masticatory muscle activity in patients with obstructive sleep apnoea. Clin Physiol Funct Imaging 2007;27(1):47–53.

115. Brown EC, Cheng S, McKenzie DK, et al. Tongue and lateral upper airway movement with mandibular advancement. Sleep 2013;36(3): 397–404.

116. Kyung SH, Park YC, Pae EK. Obstructive sleep apnea patients with oral appliance experience pharyngeal size and shape changes in three dimensions. Angle Orthod 2005;75:15–22.

117. Tsuiki S, Lowe AA, Almeida FR, et al. Effects of an anteriorly titrated mandibular position on the awake airway and obstructive sleep apnea severity. Am J Orthod Dentofacial Orthop 2004; 125:5458–555.

118. Mehta A, Qian J, Petocz P, et al. A randomized, controlled study of a mandibular advancement splint for obstructive sleep apnea. Am J Respir Crit Care Med 2001;163(6):1457–61.

119. Cooke M, Battagel JM. A thermoplastic advancement device for the management of non-apnoeic snoring: a randomized controlled trial. Eur J Orthod 2006;28(4):327–38.

120. Bartolucci ML, Bortolotti F, Raffaelli E, et al. The effectiveness of different mandibular advancement amounts in OSA patients: a systematic review and meta-regression analysis. Sleep Breath 2016;20(3): 911–9.

121. Anitua E, Durán-Cantolla J, Almeida GZ, et al. Minimizing the mandibular advancement in an oral appliance for the treatment of obstructive sleep apnea. Sleep Med 2017;34:226–31.

122. De Becker JW, Vanderveken OM, Vos WG, et al. Functional imaging using computational fluid dynamics to predict treatment success of mandibular advancement devices in sleep-disordered breathing. J Biomech 2007;40:3708–14.

123. Fritsch KM, Iseli A, Russi EW, et al. Side effects of mandibular advancement devices for sleep apnea treatment. Am J Respir Crit Care Med 2001;164(5): 813–8.

124. Norrhem N, Nemeczek H, Marklund M. Changes in lower incisor irregularity during treatment with oral sleep apnea appliances. Sleep Breath 2017; 21(3):607–13.

125. Fransson AMC, Kowalczyk A, Isacsson G. A prospective 10-year follow-up dental cast study of patients with obstructive sleep apnoea/snoring who use a mandibular protruding device. Eur J Orthod 2017;39(5):502–8.

126. Doff MHJ, Finnema KJ, Hoekema A, et al. Long-term oral appliance therapy in obstructive sleep apnea syndrome: a controlled study on dental side effects. Clin Oral Investig 2013;17:475–82.

127. Pliska BT, Nam H, Chen H, et al. Obstructive sleep apnea and mandibular advancement splints: occlusal effects and progression of changes associated with a decade of treatment. J Clin Sleep Med 2014;10(12):1285–91.

128. Cohen-Levy J, Pételle B, Pinguet J, et al. Forces created by mandibular advancement devices in OSAS patients. Sleep Breath 2013;17(2):781–9.

129. Doff M, Veldhuis SKB, Hoekema A, et al. Long-term oral appliance therapy in obstructive sleep apnea syndrome: a controlled study on temporomandibular side effects. Clin Oral Investig 2012;16(3): 689–97.

130. Nishigawa K, Hayama R, Matsuka Y. Complications causing patients to discontinue using oral appliances for treatment of obstructive sleep apnea. J Prosthodont Res 2017;61(2):133–8.

131. Sheats RD, Schell TG, Blanton AO, et al. Management of side effects of oral appliance therapy for sleep disordered breathing. J Dent Sleep Med 2017;4(4):111–25.

132. Vanderveken OM, Devolder A, Marklund M, et al. Comparison of a custom-made and a thermoplastic oral appliance for the treatment of mild sleep apnea. Am J Respir Crit Care Med 2008; 178(2):197–202.

133. Quinnell TG, Bennett M, Jordan J, et al. A crossover randomized controlled trial of oral mandibular advancement devices for obstructive sleep apnoea-hypopnoea (TOMADO). Thorax 2014;69(10):938–45.

134. Friedman M, Hamilton C, Samuelson CG, et al. Compliance and efficacy of titratable thermoplastic versus custom mandibular advancement devices. Otolaryngol Head Neck Surg 2012;147(2):379–86.

135. Johal A, Haria P, Manek S, et al. Ready-made versus custom-made mandibular repositioning devices in sleep apnea: a randomized clinical trial. J Clin Sleep Med 2017;13(2):175–82.

136. Isacsson G, Fodor C, Sturebrand M. Obstructive sleep apnea treated with custom-made bibloc and monobloc oral appliances: a retrospective comparative study. Sleep Breath 2017;21(1):93–100.

137. Ghazal A, Sorichter S, Jonas I, et al. A randomized long-term study of two oral appliances for sleep apnoea treatment. J Sleep Res 2009;18(3):321–8.

138. Bishop B, Verrett R, Girvan T. A randomized crossover study comparing two mandibular repositioning appliances for treatment of obstructive sleep apnea. Sleep Breath 2014;18(1):125–31.

139. Lawton HM, Battagel JM, Kotecha B. A comparison of the Twin Block and Herbst mandibular advancement splints in the treatment of patients with obstructive sleep apnoea: a prospective study. Eur J Orthod 2005;27(1):82–90.

140. Johnston CD, Gleadhill IC, Cinnamond MJ, et al. Mandibular appliances and obstructive sleep apnoea: a randomized clinical trial. Eur J Orthod 2002;24(3):251–62.

141. Nikolopoulou M, Byraki A, Ahlberg J, et al. Oral appliance therapy versus nasal continuous positive airway pressure in obstructive sleep apnoea

syndrome: a randomised, placebo-controlled trial on self-reported symptoms of common sleep disorders and sleep-related problems. J Oral Rehabil 2017;44(6):452–60.

142. Gauthier L, Laberge L, Beaudry M, et al. Efficacy of two mandibular advancement appliances in the management of snoring and mild-moderate sleep apnea: a cross-over randomized study. Sleep Med 2009;10(3):329–36.

143. Scherr SC, Dort LC, Almeida FR, et al. Definition of an effective oral appliance for the treatment of obstructive sleep apnea and snoring: a report of the American Academy of Dental Sleep Medicine. J Dent Sleep Med 2014;1(1):39–50.

144. Pitsis AJ, Darendeliler MA, Gotsopoulos H, et al. Effect of vertical dimension on efficacy of oral appliance therapy in obstructive sleep apnea. Am J Respir Crit Care Med 2002;166:860–4.

145. Attali V, Chamereuil C, Arnulf I, et al. Predictors of long-term effectiveness to mandibular repositioning device treatment in obstructive sleep apnea patients after 1000 days. Sleep Med 2016;27-28:107–14.

146. Chung JW, Enciso R, Levendowski DJ, et al. Patients with positional versus nonpositional obstructive sleep apnea: a retrospective study of risk factors associated with apnea-hypopnea severity. Oral Surg Oral Med Oral Pathol Oral Radiol Endod 2010;110:605–10.

147. Lamont J, Baldwin DR, Hay KD, et al. Effect of two types of mandibular advancement splints on snoring and obstructive sleep apnea. Eur J Orthod 1998;20:293–7.

148. Nikolopoulou M, Naeije M, Aarab G, et al. The effect of raising the bite without mandibular protrusion on obstructive sleep apnoea. J Oral Rehabil 2011;38:643–7.

149. Norrhem N, Marklund M. An oral appliance with or without elastic bands to control mouth opening during sleep–a randomized pilot study. Sleep Breath 2016;20(3):929–38.

150. Milano F, Mutinelli S, Sutherland K, et al. Influence of vertical mouth opening on oral appliance outcome in positional obstructive sleep apnea. J Dent Sleep Med 2018;5(1):17–23.

151. Geoghegan F, Ahrens A, McGrath C, et al. An evaluation of two different mandibular advancement devices on craniofacial characteristics and upper airway dimensions of Chinese adult obstructive sleep apnea patients. Angle Orthod 2015;85:962–8.

152. Umemoto G, Yoshimura C, Aoyagi N, et al. Treatment of the two-part semi-rigid oral appliance in obstructive sleep apnea. Oral Sci Internat 2012;9(2):49–54.

153. Vezina JP, Blumen MB, Buchet I, et al. Does propulsion mechanism influence the long-term side effects of oral appliances in the treatment of sleep-disordered breathing? Chest 2011;140(5):1184–91.

154. Izci B, McDonald JP, Coleman EL, et al. Clinical audit of subjects with snoring and sleep apnoea/hypopnea syndrome fitted with mandibular repositioning splint. Respir Med 2005;99:337–46.

155. Lee CH, Kim JW, Lee HJ, et al. Determinants of treatment outcomes after use of the mandibular advancement device in patients with obstructive sleep apnea. Arch Otolaryngol Head Neck Surg 2010;136(7):677–81.

156. Sakamoto Y, Yanamoto S, Rokutanda S, et al. Predictors of obstructive sleep apnoea-hypopnea severity and oral appliance therapy efficacy by using lateral cephalometric analysis. J Oral Rehabil 2016;43:649–55.

157. Suzuki K, Nakata S, Tagaya M, et al. Prediction of oral appliance treatment outcome in obstructive sleep apnoea syndrome: a preliminary study. B-ENT 2014;10:185–91.

158. Marklund M, Stenlund H, Franklin KA. Mandibular advancement devices in 630 men and women with obstructive sleep apnea and snoring. Chest 2004;125:1270–8.

159. Prescinotto R, Haddad FLM, Fukuchi I, et al. Impact of upper airway abnormalities on the success and adherence to mandibular advancement device treatment in patients with obstructive sleep apnea syndrome. Braz J Otorhinolaryngol 2015;81(6):663–70.

160. Remmers JE, Topor Z, Grosse J, et al. A feedback-controlled mandibular positioner identifies individuals with sleep apnea who will respond to oral appliance therapy. J Clin Sleep Med 2017;13(7):871–80.

161. Guarda-Nardini L, Manfredini D, Mion M, et al. Anatomically based outcome predictors of treatment for obstructive sleep apnea with intraoral splint devices: a systematic review of cephalometric studies. J Clin Sleep Med 2015;11(11):1327–34.

162. Neelapu BC, Kharbanda OP, Sardana HK, et al. Craniofacial and upper airway morphology in adult obstructive sleep apnea patients: a systematic review and meta-analysis of cephalometric studies. Sleep Med Rev 2017;31:79–90.

163. Sanner BM, Heise M, Knoben B, et al. MRI of the pharynx and treatment efficacy of a mandibular advancement device in obstructive sleep apnoea syndrome. Eur Respir J 2002;20:143–50.

164. Wang C-C, Chuang H-C, Hsiao H-T, et al. Applying computational fluid dynamics to optimize adjustments on oral appliance used for the treatment of snoring and sleep apnea. Sleep Med 2017;40:e3–185.

165. Zhao M, Barber T, Cistulli P, et al. Computational fluid dynamics for the assessment of upper airway response to oral appliance treatment in obstructive sleep apnea. J Biomech 2013;46:142–50.

166. Sasao Y, Nohara K, Okuno K, et al. Videoendo-scopic diagnosis for predicting the response to oral appliance therapy in severe obstructive sleep apnea. Sleep Breath 2014;18:809–15.

167. Ng AT, Qian J, Cistulli PA. Oropharyngeal collapse predicts treatment response with oral appliance therapy in obstructive sleep apnea. Sleep 2006; 29(5):666–71.

168. Johal A, Battagel JM, Kotecha BT. Sleep nasendo-scopy: a diagnostic tool for predicting treatment success with mandibular advancement splints in obstructive sleep apnoea. Eur J Orthod 2005;27: 607–14.

169. Friedman M, Shinowske K, Hamilton C, et al. Mandibular advancement for obstructive sleep apnea relating outcomes to anatomy. JAMA Otolaryngol Head Neck Surg 2014;140(1): 46–51.

170. Lee GS, Kim HK, Kim ME. Risk factors for the effi-cacy of oral appliance for treating obstructive sleep apnea: a preliminary study. Cranio 2017;8:1–8.

171. Cunha TCA, Guimarães TDM, Schultz TCB, et al. Predictors of success for mandibular repositioning appliance in obstructive sleep apnea syndrome. Braz Oral Res 2017;31:e37.

172. Landry SA, Joosten SA, Eckert DJ, et al. Therapeu-tic CPAP level predicts upper airway collapse in patients with obstructive sleep apnea. Sleep 2017;40(6). https://doi.org/10.1093/sleep/zsx056.

173. Tsuiki S, Kobayashi M, Namba K, et al. Optimal positive airway pressure predicts oral appliance response to sleep apnoea. Eur Respir J 2010; 35(5):1098–105.

174. Sutherland K, Phillips CL, Davies A, et al. CPAP pressure for prediction of oral appliance treatment response in obstructive sleep apnea. J Clin Sleep Med 2014;10:934–9.

175. Dort LC, Savard N, Dort E, et al. Does CPAP pres-sure predict outcome with oral appliances? J Dent Sleep Med 2016;3(4):113–7.

176. Storesund A, Jahansson A, Bjorvatn B, et al. Oral appliance treatment outcome can be predicted by continuous positive airway pressure in moder-ate to severe obstructive sleep apnea. Sleep Breath 2018;22(2):385–92.

177. Genta PR, Sands SA, Butler JP, et al. Airflow shape is associated with the pharyngeal structure causing OSA. Chest 2017;152(3):537–46.

178. Kuna ST, Giarrapto PC, Stanton DC, et al. Evalua-tion of an oral mandibular advancement titration appliance. Oral Surg Oral Med Oral Pathol Oral Ra-diol Endod 2006;101:593–603.

179. Sutherland K, Ngaim J, Cistulli PA. Performance of remotely controlled mandibular protrusion sleep studies for prediction of oral appliance treatment response. J Clin Sleep Med 2017; 13(3):411–7.

180. Yoshida K. Influence of sleep position on response to oral appliance therapy for sleep apnea syn-drome. Sleep 2001;24(5):538–44.

181. Lee S-A, Paek J-H, Chung Y-S, et al. Clinical fea-tures in patients with positional obstructive sleep apnea according to subtypes. Sleep Breath 2017; 21(1):109–17.

182. Ramar K, Dort L, Katz S, et al. Clinical practice guidelines for the treatment of obstructive sleep apnea and snoring with oral appliance therapy: an update for 2015. J Dent Sleep Med 2015;2(3): 71–125.

183. Engleman H, Wild MR. Improving CPAP use by pa-tients with the sleep apnea/hypopnea syndrome (SAHS). Sleep Med Rev 2003;7(1):81–9.

184. Haviv Y, Bachar G, Aframian DJ, et al. A 2-year mean follow-up of oral appliance therapy for severe obstructive sleep apnea: a cohort study. Oral Dis 2015;21:386–92.

185. Jauhar S, Lyons MF, Banham SW, et al. Ten-year follow-up of mandibular advancement devices for the management of snoring and sleep-apnea. J Prosthet Dent 2008;99:314–21.

186. McGown AD, Makker HK, Battagel JM, et al. Long-term use of mandibular advancement splints for snoring and obstructive sleep apnoea: a question-naire survey. Eur Respir J 2001;17:462–6.

187. Haviv Y, Zini A, Almozlino G, et al. Assessment of interfering factors in non-adherence to oral appli-ance therapy in severe sleep apnea. Oral Dis 2017;23:629–35.

188. Ingman T, Arte S, Bachour A, et al. Predicting compliance for mandible advancement splint ther-apy in 96 obstructive sleep apnea patients. Eur J Orthod 2013;35:752–7.

189. Zarhin D, Oksenberg A. Ambivalent adherence and nonadherence to continuous positive airway pressure devices: a qualitative study. J Clin Sleep Med 2017;13(2):1375–84.

190. Dieltjens M, Vanderveken OM, Van Den Bosch D, et al. Impact of type D personality on adherence to oral appliance therapy for sleep disordered breathing. Sleep Breath 2013;17:985–91.

191. Nadal N, de Batile J, Barbé F, et al. Predictors of CPAP compliance in different clinical settings: pri-mary care versus sleep unit. Sleep Breath 2018; 22(1):157–63.

192. Marchese-Ragona R, Manfredini D, Mion M, et al. Oral appliances for the treatment of obstructive sleep apnea in patients with low CPAP compliance: a long-term case series. Cranio 2014;32(4):254–9.

193. Kingshott RN, Jones DR, Taylor DR, et al. The efficacy of a novel tongue-stabilizing device on polysomno-graphic variables in sleep-disordered breathing: a pi-lot study. Sleep Breath 2002;6(2):69–76.

194. FDA website for LRK and LQZ. Available at: https:// www.accessdata.fda.gov/scripts/cdrh/cfdocs/cf

PMN/pmn.cfm?start_search=131&Center=&Panel
=&ProductCode=Irk&KNumber=&Applicant=&
DeviceName=&Type=&ThirdPartyReviewed=&
ClinicalTrials=&Decision=&DecisionDateFrom=
&DecisionDateTo=02%2F07%2F2018&IVDProducts=
&Redact510K=&CombinationProducts=&ZNumber
=&PAGENUM=10&SortColumn=dd%5Fdesc.

195. Canto G, Pachêco-Pereira C, Aydinoz S, et al. Diagnostic capability of biological markers in assessment of obstructive sleep apnea: a systematic review and meta-analysis. J Clin Sleep Med 2015;11(1):27–36.

196. Khalyfa A, Gileles-Hillel A, Gozol D. The challenges of precision medicine in obstructive sleep apnea. Sleep Med Clin 2016;11:213–26.

197. Sánchez-de-la-Torre M, Khalyfa A, Sánchez-de-la-Torre A, et al. Precision medicine in patients with resistant hypertension and obstructive sleep apnea. J Am Coll Cardiol 2015;66:1023–32.

198. Barbé F, Durán-Cantolla J, Sánchez-de-la-Torre M, et al. Effect of continuous positive airway pressure on the incidence of hypertension and cardiovascular events in non-sleepy patients with obstructive sleep apnea. A randomized controlled trial. JAMA 2012; 307(20):2161–8.

199. Zhang D, Luo J, Qiao Y, et al. Continuous positive airway pressure therapy in non-sleepy patients with obstructive sleep apnea: results of a meta-analysis. J Thorac Dis 2016;8(10): 2738–47.

200. Owens RL, Edwards BA, Eckert DJ, et al. An integrative model of physiological traits can be used to predict obstructive sleep apnea and response to non positive airway pressure therapy. Sleep 2015;38(6):961–70.

201. Bamagoos AA, Sutherland K, Cistulli PA. Mandibular advancement splints. Sleep Med Clin 2016; 11(3):343–52.

Clinical Evaluation for Oral Appliance Therapy

Cameron A. Kuehne, DMD, MS

KEYWORDS

- Clinical evaluation • Oral appliance therapy • Obstructive sleep apnea • Dental sleep medicine

KEY POINTS

- Treatment with oral appliance therapy (OAT) should be preceded with proper clinical examination.
- Proper clinical examination should be inclusive and include a thorough explanation of treatment to the obstructive sleep apnea patient.
- The dental professional using OAT should have proper educational training in dental sleep medicine.

INTRODUCTION

The clinical evaluation of the obstructive sleep apnea (OSA) patient to enter into oral appliance therapy (OAT) treatment is an extremely important beginning step that must be done properly to have predictable and excellent outcomes. The dentist should be confident in the areas discussed in this article and be fully able to address the needs and concerns of the OSA patient.

DISCUSSION

What Should Be Included in a Proper Clinical Evaluation for the Obstructive Sleep Apnea Patient?

Proper clinical evaluation for OAT to treat OSA is an important step in the overall process of treating the OSA patient. There are multiple criteria that should be included in a proper clinical evaluation for the patient already diagnosed with OSA that include but are not necessarily limited to the following:

- Review pertinent health history with the patient.
- Discuss the sleep study results with the patient.
- Discuss potential consequences of untreated OSA.
- Verify the patient is a good candidate for OAT with proper clinical examination.

- Obtain and discuss panoramic radiograph evaluation (or other appropriate imaging) with the patient.
- Obtain a maximum opening measurement.
- Obtain an overjet measurement.
- Obtain an overbite measurement.
- Obtain a maximum protrusion movement.
- Obtain a dental midline measurement.
- Obtain right and left lateral movement measurements.
- Note molar relationship angle.
- Note any malocclusions.
- Note any tooth wear patterns, missing teeth, or if any dental work is needed.
- Note presence of tori.
- Note tongue abnormalities related to OSA.
- Note nasal abnormalities.
- Note Mallampati score.
- Note abnormal tonsils.
- Note abnormal uvula.
- Note periodontal condition.
- Perform a temporomandibular (TM) joint palpation examination.
- Discuss OAT options and which appliance to use based on specific examination results.
- Explain the OAT titration process.
- Discuss other treatment options for OSA, such as continuous positive airway pressure (CPAP) or surgery.

8119 West Ustick Road, Boise, ID 83709, USA
E-mail address: kuehnecam@yahoo.com

Sleep Med Clin 13 (2018) 489–501
https://doi.org/10.1016/j.jsmc.2018.08.003
1556-407X/18/© 2018 Elsevier Inc. All rights reserved.

SLEEP SCREENING QUESTIONNAIRE

This questionnaire was designed to provide important facts regarding the history of your sleep condition. To assist in determining the source of any problem, please take your time and answer each question as completely and honestly as possible.

PATIENT INFORMATION

☐ MR.   ☐ MRS.   ☐ MISS   ☐ MS.   ☐ DR.   Today's Date:_____

NAME:_____
　　　　　FIRST　　　　　　　　　　MIDDLE INITIAL　　　　　　　　　LAST

ADDRESS:_____CITY/STATE/ZIP:_____

HOME PHONE:_____BUSINESS PHONE:_____ ☐ MALE ☐ FEMALE

CELL PHONE: _____ E-MAIL ADDRESS: _____

SOCIAL SECURITY NUMBER: ____-___-_____ DATE OF BIRTH: ___/___/____ AGE:_____

RESPONSIBLE PARTY:_____PHONE:_____

ADDRESS:_____CITY/STATE/ZIP:_____

EMPLOYER:_____ADDRESS:_____

REFERRED BY:_____ADDRESS:_____

FAMILY PHYSICIAN:_____ADDRESS:_____

FAMILY DENTIST:_____ADDRESS:_____

PRIMARY INSURANCE: _____   SECONDARY INSURANCE: _____
POLICY HOLDER: _____   POLICY HOLDER: _____
POLICY HOLDER DOB: _____   POLICY HOLDER DOB: _____

☐ Please check box if you are pregnant or think you might be, and let our office know.

WHAT ARE THE CHIEF COMPLAINTS FOR WHICH YOU ARE SEEKING TREATMENT?
Please number the complaints with #1 being the most important or bothersome to you.

_____ Frequent heavy snoring	_____ I have been told that "I stop breathing" when sleeping
_____ Snoring that affects the sleep of others	_____ Feeling un-refreshed in the morning
_____ Sleep apnea	_____ Morning hoarseness
_____ CPAP intolerance	_____ Morning headaches
_____ Significant daytime drowsiness	_____ Nocturnal teeth grinding
_____ Difficulty falling asleep	_____ Jaw pain
_____ Gasping when waking up	_____ Facial pain
_____ Nighttime choking spells	_____ Jaw clicking
_____ Swelling in ankles or feet	Would you be interested in a consult for Invisalign style braces? Yes ☐ No ☐

Office Use Only:
____ °F
BP:_____
Pulse: _____
Height: _____
Weight: _____

Other: _____

Patient Name _____ Date _____

Fig. 1. Sleep screening questionnaire. (*Courtesy of* Nierman Practice Management; with permission.)

- Obtain informed consent and explain potential side-effects from OAT and how to avoid side-effects.
- Obtain high-quality vinyl polysiloxane or digital impressions along with protrusive and habitual bite records.
- Obtain photographs of pretreatment condition (optional).

Review of Health History with the Patient

Health history is among the first, if not the first, item that should be discussed with the OSA patient (**Fig. 1**). **Fig. 1** shows an example of proper health history paperwork, which should be inclusive. The dentist should review the intake paperwork in depth and discuss anything related to the OSA disorder. Health history forms should, at the least, include

- Blood pressure, pulse, height, weight
- Chief complaint

- Epworth Sleepiness Scale
- Snoring, tiredness, observed apnea, blood pressure, body mass index, age, neck circumference, and gender (STOP-BANG) questionnaire
- Known allergies
- Current medications
- Medical and dental history
- Family medical history
- CPAP usage or reason for failure
- Other OSA treatment options
- Social history.

Discuss Sleep Study Results with the Patient

Often, the patient does not remember the sleep study results or has not had the results explained thoroughly. It is helpful for the patient to understand what the medical terms associated with an OSA diagnosis mean. Ideally, the dentist should explain terms such as apnea-hypopnea index

Patient Name: _____   Height: _____   Weight: _____

Epworth Sleepiness Scale

How likely are you to doze off or fall asleep in the following situations, in contrast to just feeling tired?

    0 = I would never doze   **2** = I have a moderate chance of dozing

    1 = I have a slight chance of dozing   **3** = I have a high chance of dozing

Situation   **Chance of Dozing**

1. Sitting and reading   _____
2. Watching TV   _____
3. Sitting inactive in a public place (eg, a theatre or a meeting)   _____
4. As a passenger in a car for an hour without a break   _____
5. Lying down to rest in the afternoon when circumstances permit _____
6. Sitting and talking to someone   _____
7. Sitting quietly after lunch without alcohol   _____
8. In a car while stopped for a few minutes in traffic   _____

                                  Total Score _____

		Yes	No	Not Sure
1.	Have you been told (or noticed on your own) that you snore most nights?	☐	☐	☐
2.	Have you been told (or noticed on your own) that you stop breathing or struggle to breathe in your sleep, sometimes followed by a GASP?	☐	☐	☐
3.	Are you tired, fatigued or sleepy on most days?	☐	☐	☐
4.	Do you have acid indigestion or high blood pressure (or use medication to control either of these conditions)?	☐	☐	☐
5.	Are you overweight?	☐	☐	☐
6.	Have you ever been diagnosed with obstructive sleep apnea (OSA)?	☐	☐	☐
7.	Are you currently being treated for OSA?	☐	☐	☐
8.	Are you aware of family history of OSA?	☐	☐	☐
9.	Are you aware of clenching or grinding your teeth at night?	☐	☐	☐
10.	Do you snore loudly (louder than talking or loud enough to be heard behind a closed door)?	☐	☐	☐
11.	Do you often feel tired, fatigued or sleepy during daytime?	☐	☐	☐
12.	Has anyone observed you stop breathing during your sleep?	☐	☐	☐
13.	Do you have or are you being treated for high blood pressure?	☐	☐	☐
14.	Are you 50 y old or older?	☐	☐	☐
15.	Does your neck measure more than 15 ¾ in (40 cm) around?	☐	☐	☐
16.	Are you a male?	☐	☐	☐
17.	Do you weigh more for your height than is shown in the table below?	☐	☐	☐

Height	Weight (lb)	Height	Weight (lb)	Height	Weight (lb)	Height	Weight (lb)
4'10"	167	5'3"	197	5'8"	230	6'1"	265
4'11"	173	5'4"	204	5'9"	237	6'2"	272
5'	179	5'5"	210	5'10"	243	6'3"	279
5'1"	185	5'6"	216	5'11"	250	6'4"	287
5'2"	191	5'7"	223	6'	258	6'5"	295
			Weights shown in the tables above correspond to BMI of 35 for a given height.				

Fig. 1. (*Continued*)

(including the difference between obstructive apneas vs hypopneas), sleep architecture (including the need for proper amounts of deep sleep and rapid eye movement sleep), hypoxia, and any other terms the patient may not understand. The dentist should also explain the thresholds that are within normal limits versus what is abnormal.

Discuss Potential Consequences of Untreated Obstructive Sleep Apnea

Untreated OSA is directly related to many health issues such as hypertension, stroke, heart failure, early-onset dementia, type II diabetes, Parkinson, Alzheimer, excessive daytime sleepiness, cancer, and more.[1–9] Untreated OSA has also been linked to a higher incidence of motor vehicle accidents.[10] The patient must be made aware of these concerns so that she or he is more likely become invested in treatment. Too often, the patient is diagnosed with OSA and then put on some form of treatment without being told the importance of why the treatment is needed. Explaining the potential consequences of untreated OSA may be the difference between the patient using or not using the treatment.

Verify the Patient Is a Good Candidate for Oral Appliance Therapy with Proper Clinical Examination

Before the patient can start OAT treatment, a proper clinical examination must be performed to verify the patient is a good candidate for OAT. The purpose of this examination has some important aspects. One reason is it will aid in choosing the most appropriate style of oral appliance for a specific patient. Another reason is to have good baseline records on file in the case the patient has future concerns about maxillomandibular region changes due to OAT.

LIST ANY MEDICATIONS/SUBSTANCES WHICH HAVE CAUSED YOU TO HAVE AN ALLERGIC REACTION:

_____

_____

_____

LIST ANY MEDICATIONS <u>AND</u> DOSAGE CURRENTLY BEING TAKEN (including over the counter medications, vitamins, and supplements) AND REASON FOR TAKING THE MEDICATION:

_____

_____

_____

_____

_____

MEDICAL HISTORY

Y☐ N☐ Adenoids removed	Y☐ N☐ Hay fever	Y☐ N☐ Morning dry mouth
Y☐ N☐ Tonsils removed	Y☐ N☐ Heart disorder	Y☐ N☐ Muscle spasms or cramps
Y☐ N☐ Anemia	Y☐ N☐ Heart murmur	Y☐ N☐ Muscular dystrophy
Y☐ N☐ Arteriosclerosis	Y☐ N☐ Heart pounding or beating	Y☐ N☐ Needing extra pillows to help
Y☐ N☐ Asthma	Irregularly during the night	breathing at night
Y☐ N☐ Autoimmune disorders	Y☐ N☐ Heart pacemaker	Y☐ N☐ Nervous system irritability
Y☐ N☐ Bleeding easily	Y☐ N☐ Heart palpitations	Y☐ N☐ Nighttime sweating
Y☐ N☐ Chronic sinus problems	Y☐ N☐ Heart valve replacement	Y☐ N☐ Osteoarthritis
Y☐ N☐ Chronic fatigue	Y☐ N☐ Heartburn or a sour taste in the	Y☐ N☐ Osteoporosis
Y☐ N☐ Congestive heart failure	mouth at night	Y☐ N☐ Poor circulation
Y☐ N☐ Current pregnancy	Y☐ N☐ Hepatitis	Y☐ N☐ Prior orthodontic treatment
Y☐ N☐ Depression	Y☐ N☐ High blood pressure	Y☐ N☐ Recent excessive weight gain
Y☐ N☐ Diabetes	Y☐ N☐ Immune system disorder	Y☐ N☐ Rheumatic fever
Y☐ N☐ Difficulty concentrating	Y☐ N☐ Injury to face	Y☐ N☐ Rheumatoid arthritis
Y☐ N☐ Dizziness	Y☐ N☐ Injury to mouth	Y☐ N☐ Shortness of breath
Y☐ N☐ Emphysema	Y☐ N☐ Injury to neck	Y☐ N☐ Stroke
Y☐ N☐ Epilepsy	Y☐ N☐ Injury to teeth	Y☐ N☐ Swollen, stiff, or painful joints
Y☐ N☐ Fibromyalgia	Y☐ N☐ Irregular heart beat	Y☐ N☐ TMJ disorder
Y☐ N☐ Frequent cough	Y☐ N☐ Jaw joint surgery	Y☐ N☐ Thyroid problems
Y☐ N☐ Frequent sore throat	Y☐ N☐ Low blood pressure	Y☐ N☐ Wisdom teeth extraction
Y☐ N☐ Gastroesophageal Reflux	Y☐ N☐ Memory loss	
Disease (GERD)	Y☐ N☐ Migraines	

Y☐ N☐ Other medical/dental history _____

_____

_____

_____

Patient Name _____   Date _____

Fig. 1. (_Continued_)

Obtain and Discuss Panoramic Radiograph Evaluation with the Patient

Some form of imaging is needed to evaluate the associated structures involved when treating the OSA patient. A panoramic radiograph will suffice in most cases, although computed tomography (CT) scan or MRI may be indicated based on abnormalities found on the panoramic radiograph or while performing the clinical examination. Areas to evaluate on the panoramic radiograph include the maxillary sinuses, the TM joints, the teeth, and the periodontium. Explaining the findings from the review of the imaging is an important step because it aids understanding of how anatomy is a determining factor in choosing a certain style of appliance specifically for the patient.

Obtain a Maximum Opening Measurement

An interincisal maximum opening should be taken from the incisal edge of the lower anterior teeth to the incisal edge of the upper anterior teeth (**Fig. 2**). If anterior teeth are missing, then the next most anterior teeth available to use for measurement will suffice; however, it is important to make note

FAMILY HISTORY

Do you have a loved one that has been diagnosed with obstructive sleep apnea and is not currently being treated?   Y☐ N☐

Do you have a loved one you think might have undiagnosed sleep apnea?   Y☐ N☐

Have any members of your family (blood kin) had: Y☐ N☐ Heart disease
                                                          Y☐ N☐ High blood pressure
                                                          Y☐ N☐ Diabetes

SLEEP CENTER EVALUATION

Have you ever had an evaluation at a Sleep Center?   Y ☐   N ☐

Sleep Center Name _____Location_____ Date of Study _____

CPAP (Continuous Positive Airway Pressure device)

Have you used CPAP? Y☐ N☐ For how long: _____
If you have attempted treatment with a CPAP device, but could not tolerate it please fill in this section:
          I could not tolerate the CPAP device due to: (mark all that apply)
                    _____Mask leaks
                    _____I was unable to get the mask to fit properly
                    _____Discomfort caused by the strap or headgear
                    _____Disturbed or interrupted sleep caused by the presence of the device
                    _____Noise from the device disturbing my and/or bed partner's sleep
                    _____CPAP restricted movements during sleep
                    _____CPAP does not seem to be effective
                    _____Pressure on the upper lip causing tooth related problems
                    _____A latex allergy
                    _____Claustrophobic associations
                    _____An unconscious need to remove the CPAP apparatus at night
                    _____Other: _____

OTHER THERAPY ATTEMPTS

What other therapies have you had for breathing disorders (weight loss, smoking cessation, surgery, etc.)?
_____
_____

Has any doctor recommended that you have surgery for this condition? Y☐ N☐

SOCIAL HISTORY

How often do you consume alcohol within 2–3 hours of bedtime?
          ☐ Never   ☐ Once a week   ☐ Several days a week   ☐ Daily

How often do you take sedatives within 2–3 hours of bedtime?
          ☐ Never   ☐ Once a week   ☐ Several days a week   ☐ Daily

How often do you consume caffeine within 2–3 hours of bedtime?
          ☐ Never   ☐ Once a week   ☐ Several days a week   ☐ Daily

Do you smoke? Y ☐ N ☐   If YES, how many a day? _____
Do you use chewing tobacco? Y ☐ N ☐

Patient Name _____ Date _____

Fig. 1. (*Continued*)

of which teeth were used in taking the measurement. A normal maximum opening is between 40 mm to 60 mm without pain. If the patient opens to the acceptable range with pain or cannot open to at least 40 mm, there may be a TM disorder (TMD) issue, which should be addressed at that time.

During the opening stroke, it should be noted if the patient has a deviation or deflection of the mandible. Deviation of the mandible means that the mandible moves to 1 side during opening but returns to the midline on full opening. A deflection of the mandible means that the mandible moves to 1 side during opening and remains to the side on full opening. Both deviation and deflection could signify a potential internal derangement of 1 or both TM joints.

It is important to use a device with a 0 starting point. Note that the ruler in the figure has been shaved to remove any material so that the edge of the ruler is at the 0 hash mark (see **Fig. 2**).

Obtain an Overjet Measurement

An overjet measurement is taken by placing the ruler on the labial surface of the lower anterior

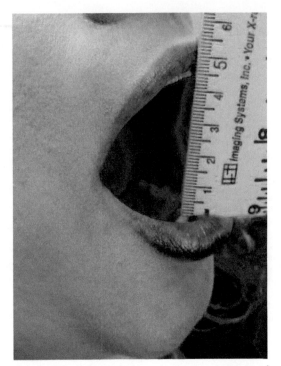

Fig. 2. This patient has a maximum opening of 45 mm.

teeth and measuring the overlap to the incisal edge of the upper anterior teeth with the patient in centric occlusion[11] (**Fig. 3**).

Obtain an Overbite Measurement

An overbite measurement is taken by having the patient close in centric occlusion and marking the point where the upper anterior teeth overlap the lower anterior teeth (**Fig. 4**).[11] The patient then opens his or her mouth and a measurement of the amount of overlap can be recorded from the marked point.

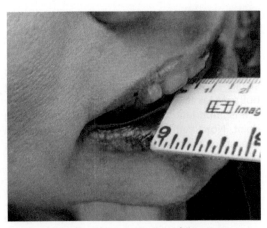

Fig. 3. This patient has an overjet of 2 mm.

Obtain a Maximum Protrusion Movement

A maximum protrusion movement is obtained by adding the overjet measurement to the maximum movement a patient can protrude the mandibular anterior teeth past the maxillary anterior teeth (**Fig. 5**). This measurement is taken by measuring from the labial surface of the upper anterior teeth to the incisal edge of the lower teeth and then adding that number to the overjet measurement. A normal maximum protrusion movement is between 8 mm to 12 mm without pain. If the protrusion is in the acceptable range but with pain or if the maximum protrusion movement is less than 8 mm, there may be a TMD issue, which should be immediately addressed.

Obtain a Dental Midline Measurement

A dental midline measurement is obtained by measuring the distance between the embrasure of the upper central incisors to the embrasure of the lower central incisors with the teeth in centric occlusion (**Fig. 6**). It is important to note any midline deviations if present. A midline that is off to 1 side by more than 4 mm is considered abnormal.

Obtain Right and Left Lateral Movement Measurements

Lateral movement measurements are recorded by having the patient move the mandible to 1 side and measuring the distance from the embrasure of the

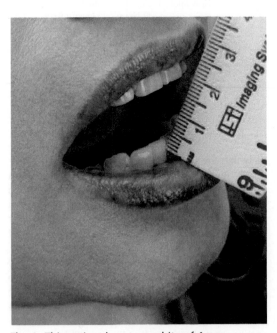

Fig. 4. This patient has an overbite of 4 mm.

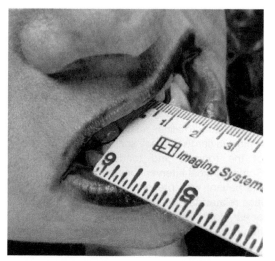

Fig. 5. This patient has a 4 mm protruded movement plus a 2 mm overjet (see **Fig. 3**) for a total maximum protrusive movement of 6 mm.

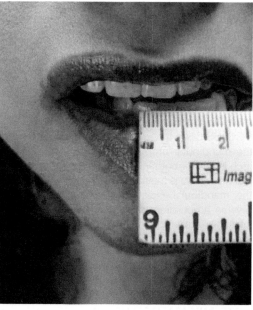

Fig. 7. This patient has a left lateral movement of 9 mm.

upper central incisors to the embrasure of the lower central incisors (**Figs. 7** and **8**). A lateral movement is between 8 mm to 12 mm without pain. If the movement is in the acceptable range but with pain or if the movement is less than 8 mm, there may be a TMD issue, which should be immediately addressed.

NOTE ANGLE MOLAR CLASSIFICATION

As defined by the "Glossary of Prosthodontic terms," "Class I (normal occlusion or NEUTRO-OCCLUSION): the dental relationship in which there is normal anteroposterior relationship of the jaws, as indicated by intercuspal position of maxillary and mandibular molars, but with crowding and rotation of teeth elsewhere, i.e., a dental dysplasia or arch length deficiency; Class II (DISTO-OCCLUSION): the dental relationship in which the mandibular dental arch is posterior to the maxillary dental arch in one or both lateral segments; the mandibular first molar is distal to the maxillary first molar; Class II can be further subdivided into two divisions; Division 1: bilateral distal retrusion with a

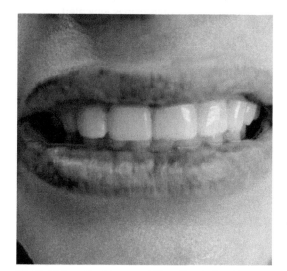

Fig. 6. This patient has a midline that is "on," or not deviated.

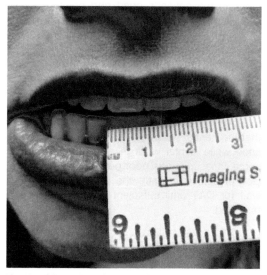

Fig. 8. This patient has a right lateral movement of 9 mm.

narrow maxillary arch and protruding maxillary incisors. Subdivisions include right or left (unilaterally distal with other characteristics being the same); Division 2: bilateral distal with a normal or square-shaped maxillary arch, retruded maxillary central incisors, labially malposed maxillary lateral incisors, and an excessive vertical overlap. Subdivisions include right or left (unilaterally distal with other characteristics the same); Class III (MESIO-OCCLUSION): the dental relationship in which the mandibular arch is anterior to the maxillary arch in one or both lateral segments; the mandibular first molar is mesial to the maxillary first molar; the mandibular incisors are usually in anterior reverse articulation; subdivisions include right or left (unilaterally mesial with other characteristics the same)."[12]

If first molars are not present, canine teeth may be used to determine if the patient has a class I, II, or III occlusion.

NOTE ANY MALOCCLUSION

Any issues such as crossbites, unstable dental contacts, tooth crowding, or tooth spacing should be noted and pointed out to the patient. This record will help the dentist in follow-up to determine if any changes have occurred in occlusal relationships. It also helps the patient to be aware of any issues before treatment is rendered.

NOTE ANY TOOTH WEAR PATTERNS, MISSING TEETH, OR IF ANY DENTAL WORK IS NEEDED

It is important to verify any parafunctional habits and on which teeth they occur. A note should be made in the patient's chart and pointed out so that the patient is aware of the tooth wear before an appliance is inserted. Tooth wear, especially from lateral movements, is a determining factor when choosing the appliance design.

It is also important to note any teeth in need of dental work. All efforts should be made to fabricate the oral appliance to protect the patient's airway as soon as possible. At times, this may mean that the dentist will need to modify the oral appliance while dental work is being completed. In some cases, such as poor periodontal support or lack of sufficient teeth, the patient will need to wait for OAT until sufficient dental treatment is rendered.

NOTE PRESENCE OF TORI

Tori are bony growths found in both the mandible and maxilla. These can cause problems in getting proper impressions to fabricate a custom oral appliance. Tori size and location should be noted in the patient's chart and care in appliance selection should be taken into account when dealing with especially large tori.

NOTE TONGUE ABNORMALITIES RELATED TO OBSTRUCTIVE SLEEP APNEA

Tongue abnormalities related to OSA include macroglossia (large tongue), scalloping on the borders of the tongue, and tongue-tie complications. Some surgical interventions may be beneficial for the patient who presents with tongue abnormalities related to OSA.[13] Referral to an oral surgeon or ear, nose, and throat (ENT) doctor for consultation may be indicated if the tongue abnormality is severe.

NOTE NASAL ABNORMALITIES RELATED TO OBSTRUCTIVE SLEEP APNEA

Nasal abnormalities related to OSA include congestion due to rhinitis or infection, deviated septum, large turbinates, large adenoids, and constricted nasal passages.[14]

Issues such as a deviated septum and large adenoids can be seen radiographically. In an ideal setting, the dentist who uses cone-beam CT for a radiologic screening tool will have a board-certified radiologist interpret the image and provide a report. This extra step will ensure that the dentist does not miss an important anatomic concern.

Other issues with the nose, such as large turbinates or constricted nasal passages, can be seen using a speculum. If this is outside of the scope of the dentist's practice, referral for consultation with an ENT physician is indicated.

NOTE MALLAMPATI SCORE

Mallampati classification is used by anesthesiologists when evaluating the airway before surgery that requires intubation[15] (**Fig. 9**). A properly done Mallampati examination is done with the patient's mouth open and tongue sticking out but not saying "ahh" because doing so tenses the soft palate and makes the airway appear more open than it would be during sleep. A class III or class IV Mallampati score is associated with a higher risk for OSA.

NOTE ABNORMAL TONSILS

A quick examination of the back of the throat allows for a view of the tonsils. Abnormally large tonsils may be of concern and referral for consult with an ENT doctor may be indicated. Note that tonsil

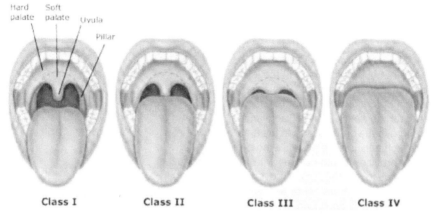

Class I   Class II   Class III   Class IV

Fig. 9. Mallampati classification. (*From* Elo J, Sun H. Anesthesia and sedation, a textbook of advanced oral and maxillofacial surgery. In: Kalantar Motamedi MH, editor. vol. 3. InTech: 2016. https://doi.org/10.5772/63539; with permission.)

size in the pediatric patient does not directly correlate to severity of OSA.[16]

NOTE ABNORMAL UVULA

An abnormal uvula will often look elongated and/or battered in appearance. This indicates a chronic sleep-disordered breathing condition.[17]

NOTE PERIODONTAL CONDITION

The periodontal condition is important. Forces applied to the periodontium due to OAT can cause concern for long-term dental health of the periodontally compromised OSA patient. If present, there should be notation of the degree and the location of the periodontal loss. If periodontal inflammation is present, the location should also be noted. These issues should be brought to the patient's attention before starting treatment to raise awareness of the existing problem so that the patient can actively do something about his or her periodontal health.

Again, all measures should be taken to treat the patient and protect the airway in a timely manner; however, if the periodontium is too compromised, the patient may need to seek dental treatment before OAT treatment is practical.

PERFORM A TEMPOROMANDIBULAR JOINT PALPATION EXAMINATION

TM joint palpation can be done by placing the fingers slightly anterior to the tragus of the ear and having the patient open and close the mouth and by moving the mandible laterally. Alternatively, auscultation may be done with a stethoscope. If any clicking or popping is felt or heard, the patient most likely has an internal derangement of the TM

joint. Proper documentation of the derangement should include on which side the derangement occurred or if it was bilateral. It should also be noted if the click or pop was an early, middle, or late pop in the opening stroke. An important point is that an internal derangement of the TM joint does not preclude the patient from OAT treatment, even if the patient has current TM joint pain. It is, however, important for the dentist to thoroughly explain the condition and to be able to properly guide the patient through treatment with an oral appliance. It is highly recommended that the dentist have a thorough understanding of treating TMD side effects from use of OAT.

DISCUSS ORAL APPLIANCE THERAPY OPTIONS AND WHICH APPLIANCE TO USE BASED ON SPECIFIC EXAMINATION RESULTS

Currently, there is not a custom, titratable oral appliance that works for every patient. There are too many variables for a specific oral appliance to always be the best option. No current literature has proven that any custom, titratable oral appliance is superior from an efficacy standpoint. Therefore, the dentist should have knowledge of multiple custom, titratable oral appliance options for the patient. A custom, titratable appliance should be used long-term instead of an option that is not custom or titratable.[18]

Of the many styles of oral appliances that are currently approved by the US Food and Drug Administration, most fit into 1 of 4 categories: push, pull, interlocking, and anterior point stop appliances. Each category has positives and negatives. A proper clinical examination of the OSA patient will help the dentist to make a decision that is best for the patient.

Push Appliances

Push appliances are good for people with missing lower posterior teeth (**Fig. 10**). Due to the forces on the lower anterior teeth, special care must be taken to assure that the periodontium in the lower anterior region can bear such forces. These types of appliances can be difficult to adjust for people with poor manual dexterity. These appliances can be bothersome to the oral mucosa in the areas of the titration mechanisms. The patient who presents with lateral bruxism would do well with this style of appliance due to the freedom of movement laterally. The claustrophobic patient or the patient who sleeps with the mouth open can do well with this style of oral appliance.

Pull Appliances

Pull appliances are good for people with missing upper posterior teeth (**Fig. 11**). Due to the forces on the upper anterior teeth, special care must be taken to assure that the periodontium in the upper anterior region can bear such forces. These types of appliances may be less difficult to adjust for people with poor manual dexterity. These appliances can be bothersome to the oral mucosa in the areas of the titration mechanisms. The patient who presents with lateral bruxism would do well with this style of appliance (with most styles in this category) due to the freedom of movement laterally. The claustrophobic patient or the patient who sleeps with the mouth open can do well with this style of oral appliance, although a push or interlocking style appliance may be better tolerated.

Interlocking Appliances

Interlocking appliances are good for people with minimal retentive features due to the upper and lower pieces not being connected to each other (**Fig. 12**). Forces tend to be concentrated on the

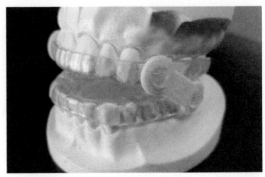

Fig. 11. The EMA design is an example of a pull appliance. (*Courtesy of* Myerson Tooth Company, Chicago, IL; with permission.)

premolar and molar regions. These types of appliances can be difficult to adjust for people with poor manual dexterity. The patient who presents with lateral bruxism is not an ideal candidate for this style of appliance (although there are some exceptions). The claustrophobic patient or the patient who sleeps with the mouth open, should do well with these styles of appliances.

Anterior Point Stop Appliances

Anterior point stop appliances are good for people missing posterior teeth due to the forces being concentrated on the anterior teeth (**Fig. 13**). Due to the forces on the anterior teeth, special care must be taken to assure that the periodontium in the anterior region can bear such forces. These types of appliances can be difficult to adjust for people with poor manual dexterity. These appliances can also reduce tongue space due to the titration mechanism being location anteriorly. The patient who presents with lateral bruxism would do well with this style of appliance due to the freedom of movement laterally. The claustrophobic patient or the patient who sleeps with the

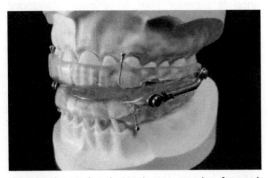

Fig. 10. The Herbst design is an example of a push appliance.

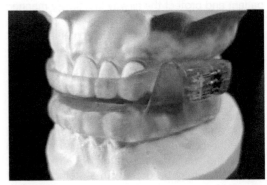

Fig. 12. The Dorsal Fin design is an example of an interlocking appliance.

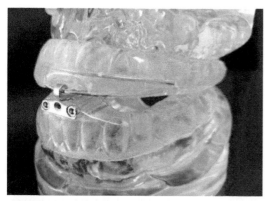

Fig. 13. The DreamTAP design is an example of an anterior point stop appliance. (*Courtesy of* Airway Labs out of Carrollton, TX; with permission.)

mouth open, may not do well with these styles of oral appliances.

An important note for dentists working with medical insurance is to understand the rules of the insurance companies. Some companies mandate that certain appliances be used for the OSA patient to have the OAT treatment covered.

EXPLAIN THE ORAL APPLIANCE THERAPY TITRATION PROCESS

After an appliance is chosen based on proper clinical examination, it is important to explain the OAT titration process, both the mechanism of adjustment and the subjective findings associated with improvement during the process. Ideally, the patient will be able to handle a model of the appliance at this point to experience the feel of adjusting the titration mechanism. After this has been covered, a discussion of the purpose of titrating the appliance to find the best treatment position should include explanation of the criteria of subjective improvement. It may also be a good time to explain that further protrusion of the mandible is not necessarily always better. An explanation of the purpose

---

Informed Consent for the Treatment of Sleep Disordered Breathing

You have been diagnosed by your physician as requiring treatment for sleep-disordered breathing (snoring and/or obstructive sleep apnea). This condition may pose serious health risks since it disrupts normal sleep patterns and can reduce normal blood oxygen levels, which in turn, may result in the following: excessive daytime sleepiness, irregular heartbeats, high blood pressure, heart attack or stroke.

What Is Oral Appliance Therapy?

Oral appliance therapy for snoring/obstructive sleep apnea attempts to assist breathing during sleep by keeping the tongue and jaw in a forward position during sleeping hours. Oral appliance therapy has effectively treated many patients. However, there are no guarantees that it will be effective for you, since everyone is different and there are many factors influencing the upper airway during sleep. It is important to recognize that even when the therapy is effective, there may be a period of time before the appliance functions maximally. During this time you may still experience the symptoms related to your sleep disordered breathing. A post-adjustment polysomnogram (sleep study) is necessary to objectively assure effective treatment. This must be obtained from your physician.

Side-Effects and Complications of Oral Appliance Therapy

Published studies show that short-term effects of oral appliance use may include excessive salivation, difficulty swallowing (with appliance in place), sore jaws, sore teeth, jaw joint pain, dry mouth, gum pain, loosening of teeth and short-term bite changes (how the upper and lower teeth come together). There are also reports of dislodgement of ill-fitting dental restorations and in some cases it is possible that porcelain may fracture off of crown and bridge restorations. Most of these side effects are minor and resolve quickly on their own or with minor adjustment of the appliance. Long-term complications include bite changes that may be permanent resulting from tooth movement or jaw joint repositioning. These complications may or may not be fully reversible once appliance therapy is discontinued. If not, restorative treatment or orthodontic intervention may be required for which you will be responsible.

Follow up visits with the provider of your oral appliance are mandatory to ensure proper fit and allow an examination of your mouth to assure a healthy condition. If unusual symptoms or discomfort occur that fall outside the scope of this consent, or if pain medication is required to control discomfort, it is recommended you cease using the appliance until you are evaluated further.

Alternative Treatment for Sleep Disordered Breathing

Other accepted treatments for sleep-disordered breathing include behavioral modifications, positive airway pressure and various surgeries. It is your decision to have chosen oral appliance therapy to treat your sleep disordered breathing and you are aware that it may not be completely effective for you. It is your responsibility to report the occurrence of side effects and to address any questions to this provider's office. Failure to treat sleep disordered breathing may increase the likelihood of significant medical complications.

If you have any comfort issues/concerns with your appliance CALL OUR OFFICE RIGHT AWAY! DO NOT WAIT! It is your responsibility to inform us of your concerns. There are options that we can provide to help you. If you understand the explanation of the proposed treatment, have asked this provider any questions you may have about this form or treatment, please sign and date this form below.

Print Name: _____

Signature: _____   Date: _____

Fig. 14. Informed consent form for the treatment of sleep-disordered breathing.

of proper and timely follow-up appointments at the dental office to evaluate progress should be stressed. At this point, the patient should be informed of the potential need for objective follow-up testing if requested by her or his medical doctor.

DISCUSS OTHER TREATMENT OPTIONS FOR OBSTRUCTIVE SLEEP APNEA

If the patient has not yet tried CPAP therapy, a discussion should be had about the option to use CPAP if OAT fails. This may be a good time to also talk about the possibility of combination therapy. If during the clinical examination the dentist discovers an anatomic finding contributing to the OSA diagnosis for which surgery may be a benefit, a consult to an ENT doctor or oral surgeon may be indicated.

OBTAIN INFORMED CONSENT AND EXPLAIN POTENTIAL SIDE-EFFECTS FROM ORAL APPLIANCE THERAPY AND HOW TO AVOID SIDE-EFFECTS

OAT causes side-effects. These side-effects can cause tooth movement, bite changes, and short-term TMD issues.[19] It is important to let the patient know about these potential issues and how to avoid them. Ideally, the dentist should discuss side-effects and how to avoid side-effects at every single appointment.

It is also important for the dentist to have an informed consent form stating that side-effects, along with strategies to avoid side-effects, were explained to the OSA patient (**Fig. 14**). The patient who refuses to sign informed consent should not be allowed to enter treatment.

OBTAIN HIGH-QUALITY VINYL POLYSILOXANE OR DIGITAL IMPRESSIONS ALONG WITH PROTRUSIVE AND HABITUAL BITE RECORDS

The most important step in making an oral appliance to treat OSA is the impression. A poor impression will lead to a poor outcome. The dentist must have either high-quality vinyl polysiloxane impressions or digital impressions with proper protrusive and habitual bite records. Ideally, these records should be kept for as long as the patient is in the care of the dentist so that there is a baseline of the original tooth position and the original habitual bite position.

SUMMARY

When done correctly, a proper clinical examination will lead to predictable and excellent outcomes for both the OSA patient and the treating dentist. It is suggested that the dentist be fully confident in the skills outlined in this article so that treatment is at the highest level possible. If that confidence is lacking, nonprofit or university-based continuing education courses to gain this skillset are recommended.

REFERENCES

1. Sharma S, Culebras A. Sleep apnoea and stroke. Stroke Vasc Neurol 2016;e000038. https://doi.org/10.1136/svn-2016-000038.
2. Gozal D, Farré R, Nieto FJ. Putative links between sleep apnea and cancer: from hypotheses to evolving evidence. Chest 2015;148(5):1140–7.
3. Martin R, Cowie AM. Gallagher. Sleep disordered breathing and heart failure. JACC Heart Fail 2017; 699. https://doi.org/10.1016/j.jchf.2017.06.016.
4. Doumit J, Prasad B. Sleep apnea in type 2 diabetes. Diabetes Spectr 2016;29(1):14–9.
5. Ahmad M, Makati D, Akbar S. Review of and updates on hypertension in obstructive sleep apnea. Int J Hypertens 2017;2017:1848375.
6. Emamian F, Khazaie H, Tahmasian M, et al. The association between obstructive sleep apnea and Alzheimer's disease: a meta-analysis perspective. Front Aging Neurosci 2016;8:78.
7. Chou P-S, Lai C-L, Chou Y-H, et al. Sleep apnea and the subsequent risk of Parkinson's disease: a 3-year nationwide population-based study. Neuropsychiatr Dis Treat 2017;13:959–65.
8. Rossor MN, Fox NC, Mummery CJ, et al. The diagnosis of young-onset dementia. Lancet Neurol 2010;9(8):793–806.
9. Obaseki D, Erhabor G, Obaseki J, et al. Obstructive sleep apnea, excessive daytime sleepiness, and road traffic accidents among interstate commercial vehicle drivers in Nigeria. J Respir Med 2014;2014:7.
10. De Mello MT, Narciso FV, Tufik S, et al. Sleep disorders as a cause of motor vehicle collisions. Int J Prev Med 2013;4(3):246–57.
11. Heikinheimo K, Nyström M, Heikinheimo T, et al. Dental arch width, overbite, and overjet in a Finnish population with normal occlusion between the ages of 7 and 32 years. Eur J Orthod 2012;34(4):418–26.
12. The glossary of prosthodontic terms. J Prosthet Dentist 2005;94(1):10–92.
13. Caples S, Rowley J, Prinsell J, et al. Surgical modifications of the upper airway for obstructive sleep apnea in adults: a systematic review and meta-analysis. Sleep 2010;33(10):1396–407.
14. Young T, Skatrud J, Peppard PE. Risk factors for obstructive sleep apnea in adults. JAMA 2004; 291(16):2013–6.
15. Liistro G, Rombaux P, Belge C, et al. High Mallampati score and nasal obstruction are associated

risk factors for obstructive sleep apnoea. Eur Respir J 2003;21(2):248252.

16. Nolan J, Brietzke S. Systematic review of pediatric tonsil size and polysomnogram-measured obstructive sleep apnea severity. Otolaryngol Head Neck Surg 2011;144(6):844–50.

17. Sekosan M, Zakkar M, Wenig B, et al. Inflammation in the uvula mucosa of patients with obstructive sleep apnea. Laryngoscope 1996;106:1018–20.

18. Vanderveken O, Devolder A, Marklund M, et al. Comparison of a custom-made and a thermoplastic oral appliance for the treatment of mild sleep apnea. Am J Respir Crit Care Med 2008; 178(2):197–202.

19. Fritsch K, Iseli A, Russi E, et al. Side effects of mandibular advancement devices for sleep apnea treatment. Am J Respir Crit Care Med 2001;164(5): 813–8.

Avoiding and Managing Oral Appliance Therapy Side Effects

Thomas G. Schell, DMD, DABDSM[a,b,]*

KEYWORDS

- Oral appliance therapy • Side effects of OAT • Obstructive sleep apnea • Dental sleep medicine

KEY POINTS

- There is a serious need to consider all potential side effects thoughtfully before commencing individual treatment.
- Although many of these side effects are self-limiting, easily corrected, or innocuous, others are difficult or impossible to correct and can affect the patient in some serious ways.
- If alternative treatment is not acceptable, the carefully weighed risk of no therapy is what allows practitioners to justify these likely problems to coexist with oral appliance therapy.
- As this field evolves, new information is discovered, and new products are introduced at a rather rapid pace, continuing education and prudent practice are critical to ethical care in the practice of dental sleep medicine.

INTRODUCTION

Oral appliance therapy (OAT) is being used more frequently in the management of obstructive sleep apnea (OSA) as an alternative to continuous positive air pressure. As the frequency of OAT use is increasingly more popular and as more patients are consistently adherent to it over longer periods of time, side effects from this therapy are becoming more clinically evident in both frequency and magnitude.

A *side effect* for the purpose of this article represents any untoward or unexpected outcome; one not intended and quite possibly, but not always having a deleterious effect. Side effects from OAT are common and expectable. The extent to which a side effect is intolerable to a patient is a very individual concern and will vary greatly between patients. One patient's limit for an intolerable bite change may well be within the tolerable range for another. All risks of potential side effects should be weighed against the risks of no therapy, provided no alternative treatment is acceptable.

It is critical for providers to get a broad-reaching and objective range of education in this field before commencing in the practice of dental sleep medicine (DSM). Having an understanding of the number of different side effects that potentially occur from OAT use and their ability to affect the patient in many different ways is critically important. Regular ongoing continuing education in an effort to remain abreast of the constantly evolving changes in this field is essential to be able to predict, prevent, and manage these side effects when they do occur.

There has traditionally been a large gap in knowledge regarding side effects from OAT. Most evidence is anecdotal. What limited research exists on this topic can be difficult to locate, understand, and apply in clinical practice for an average

No conflict of interest or funding sources to disclose.
[a] Dr Thomas G Schell and Dr. Patrick C Noble PLLC, 31 Old Etna Road, N1 Lebanon, NH 03770, USA;
[b] Department of Surgery, Dartmouth Geisel School of Medicine, 1 Rope Ferry Road, Hanover, NH 03755-1404, USA
* PO Box 127, Meriden, NH 03770.
E-mail address: tgschell@gmail.com

Sleep Med Clin 13 (2018) 503–512
https://doi.org/10.1016/j.jsmc.2018.07.003

practitioner. Although many of these side effects are self-limiting, easily corrected, or innocuous, others are difficult or impossible to correct and can affect the patient in some serious ways.

Recently, in an effort to bridge this informational gap, a panel of experts was convened by the American Academy of Dental Sleep Medicine (AADSM) Board of Directors to look at side effects from OAT and their management. Until that time, there had not been an analysis performed with recommendations to detail these issues for clinicians. As a key preliminary part of this process, an exhaustive literature review was performed. In addition, a comprehensive survey of a large number of highly regarded providers in the field was conducted. All of this informational data were carefully analyzed. The panel was able to identify and differentiate these various side effects as well as come to agreement on the most appropriate management of each. The consensus article was published in the October 10, 2017, issue of the *Journal of Dental Sleep Medicine*.[1]

This publication represented the first thorough set of clinical guidelines specifically related to side effects and their management. It was put forth to act as a useful reference tool for practitioners and researchers seeking guidance on the management of these issues in the clinical setting. Until such time as we can turn solely to empirical evidence on side effects, any consideration of these issues should rely on the findings of the experts' conference. This article refers to it as the standard of reference to date.

THE SIDE EFFECTS CONSENSUS CONFERENCE: OVERVIEW

Experts from across the field of DSM were selected to act as voting members on a consensus panel using the UCLA/RAND appropriateness of care method. The selected 13-member panel consisted of dentists chosen with specific intention toward their proper protocol for diagnosis, application of treatment, and follow-up of DSM as well as for their experience in temporomandibular joint (TMJ), occlusion and oral health in general.

As an initial part of the process, an exhaustive literature search and review was performed to seek all published evidence of side effects for consideration. This search resulted in 181 articles published through February 2016. A total of 143 of these were subsequently chosen to be included in the study. In addition, a rather detailed survey of the diplomats of the American Board of Dental Sleep Medicine as well as AADSM committee members was performed to seek out side effects as they presented in clinical experience for review

as well. Fifty-one percent of these surveys were returned and reviewed by the panel in addition to the literature.

With the raw data from the literature and the survey at hand, the panel was then able to consolidate the side effects into 5 categories: (1) TMJ issues, (2) problems with intraoral tissues, (3) changes in occlusion, (4) damage to teeth or restorations, and (5) various other appliance issues.

Voting on the appropriateness of each side-effect treatment within each category was accomplished anonymously via e-mail and then again after the careful review of evidence in 2 additional rounds of voting at the face-to-face conference. The RAND process definitively defines the level of agreement on each item under consideration. Only those treatments clearly deemed appropriate after review of the literature and survey results were retained for additional voting and inclusion in the final recommendations. Any treatments deemed either inappropriate or uncertain were dropped from consideration. The final vote was to qualitatively define whether each treatment represented should be considered primarily, as a second-line option, or whether it was uncommon, but still merited appropriate consideration for use by practitioners.

These methodically established recommendations were then endorsed by the AADSM Board of Directors for publication in the *Journal of Dental Sleep Medicine*. It was noted that this should not be considered an exhaustive list of choices in the management of side effects. While addressing the breadth of common side effects and their management, these recommendations should also be used with clinical expertise and judgment gained through rigorous training in DSM. These can then be adapted in the most appropriate and specific way for any given patient and situation.

CONSENT

As with any medical procedure that carries some risk for unexpected or untoward results, a detailed informed consent process is critical to ensuring both proper education to the patient and protection for the practitioner. Written informed consents should be both easy to read and understand by the average patient population. This also must be detailed enough to not miss the significant risk associated with any unwanted side effects. Most experienced practitioners will inform their patients that they will likely experience some side effects. It is the degree to which they can be tolerated that should be weighed against alternative treatment or the risk of no treatment at all. These written informed consent documents should be explained verbally and signed with a witness before beginning any treatment. One popular site in the marketplace offers 36 specific informed consent, informed-refusal, and release-of-liability documents for practitioners providing OAT; this implies the broad-reaching significance of these concerns.

PRETREATMENT RECORDS

To identify and be able to measure any side effects, it is necessary that each practitioner gather detailed pretreatment records of the patient in both anatomic position and function. This would take the form of (but is not necessarily limited to) cast models, photos of the patient's occlusion in habitual position, and a physical bite record. Additionally, pretreatment measurements of overjet and overbite, interproximal contacts, and interocclusal contacts using thin shim stock would be important to have on record in any ongoing evaluation of potential changes. Finally, pretreatment assessment of the TMJ and muscles of the head and neck as well as the periodontium also should be recorded. These can include records of maximum interincisal opening, both lateral and anterior excursion, as well as qualitative objective evaluation of the joint using visual and bimanual palpation. Audio analysis can be useful as well, using stethoscope and/or Doppler ultrasound. Deviations or shifts in both the path of opening and closing, carefully noting any clicks, pops, and crepitus also can be helpful if evaluating changes in comfort or function during treatment. Preoperative radiographic imaging of the TMJ is also important as a tool to rule out disease and potentially uncover any pathologic change over the course of treatment.

RECALL AND FOLLOW-UP

It is very important to discover progressive side effects early to have the best chance to correct them, or at least to limit their negative effect. This requires early and frequent recall initially and regular follow-up thereafter; on a frequency of at least once per year unless there have been signs of changes that would warrant more frequent evaluation. Any side effect encountered must be detailed in its effect, its management, and throughout its resolution. Here is where baseline records are indispensable. Any side effect must be immediately disclosed to the patient and a detailed discussion of all conceivable consequences of such a change take place. If the decision is made with the patient to discontinue OAT, then alternative treatment options should then be discussed with

the patient and documented. In this instance, communication with, and referral back to the managing physician is necessary to be sure that the patient does not go without care. This also needs to be documented in the patient record.

The various different side effects identified by the panelists at the consensus conference are listed in **Box 1**. These side effects were each defined and management protocol was explained for each in the publication.

In addition to the specific management plan recommended by the experts, there were a number of common management considerations that had a broad-reaching application to many if not all of

---

Box 1
Side effects

Temporomandibular joint–related side effects
- Transient morning jaw pain
- Persistent temporomandibular joint pain
- Tenderness in muscles of mastication
- Joint sounds

Intraoral tissue–related side effects
- Soft tissue and tongue irritation
- Gingival irritation
- Excessive salivation/drooling
- Dry mouth

Occlusal changes
- Altered occlusal contacts/bite changes
- Incisor changes
- Decreased overjet and overbite
- Alterations in positions of mandibular canines and molars
- Interproximal gaps

Damage to teeth or restorations
- Tooth mobility
- Tooth fractures or damage to dental restorations

Appliance issues
- Appliance breakage
- Allergies to appliance material
- Gagging
- Anxiety

From Sheats RD, Schell TG, Blanton AO, et al. Management of side effects of oral appliance therapy for sleep disordered breathing. J Dent Sleep Med 2017; 4(4):113; with permission.

these side effects. These follow here as choices that should be considered in many common circumstances and will be listed out individually again in each of the specific side-effect recommendations where they apply.

COMMON MANAGEMENT CONSIDERATIONS
Palliative Care

"Palliative care is supportive in nature and intended to manage patient discomfort during the healing phase. It may include any/all of the following options: reassurance, rest, ice, soft diet, topical or systemic pain relief products or anti-inflammatory medications, massage, and physiotherapy."[1]

Watchful Waiting

"Watchful waiting is the ongoing process of careful and diligent observation, with the possibility of additional assessment along the way, in an effort to better understand the side-effect process. Documentation of the process must be included in the patient's record and follow-up of concerns at subsequent visits should occur and be recorded regarding persistence, resolution or management of side effects."[1]

Morning Occlusal Guide

"Morning occlusal guide encompasses many custom-made appliances and prefabricated devices used in the effort to reposition the mandible into its habitual pretreatment position. These devices may function by using biting forces to reseat the condyles to help reestablish/maintain the appropriate occlusal relationship in the morning following each night of OAT. Some of these custom devices may function by reversing changes that may have occurred in tooth position or work to exercise or stretch muscles of mastication as well. They are intended to address the occlusal discrepancy noted after removal of the appliance each morning."[1]

"Before the patient begins using the oral appliance, the morning occlusal guide is fabricated chair-side or by a laboratory, and is often made of hard acrylic, thermoplastic, or compressible materials. The guide must be adapted to the patient's maxillary and mandibular teeth in habitual occlusion or to dental casts in maximum intercuspation."[1]

"Intended to address the occlusal discrepancy noted after the removal of the oral appliance each morning, morning occlusal guides also help patients to monitor their condition by allowing them to ascertain whether their mandible is correctly aligned every morning. Each morning after the sleep appliance is worn, the patient should bite into the guide until the maxillary and mandibular teeth are fully seated for as long as it takes the teeth to reestablish occlusion. In the event that the patient is unable to attain proper habitual occlusion, the patient should contact the oral appliance provider."[1]

It is important to note that despite widespread use of morning repositioners or occlusal guides, there is no clinical evidence that links these with any specific success at either preventing or managing side effects of OAT.

Daytime Intraoral Orthotic

"The daytime intraoral orthotic encompasses many custom appliances and prefabricated devices that are retained by either the maxillary or mandibular dentition/implants. These devices are intended to deprogram masticatory muscles, reseat the mandibular condyles, and/or reduce the magnitude and frequency of bruxism events as well as its consequences. Distinctive from the morning occlusal guide, this device is intended for more active therapy of preexisting or iatrogenically created conditions affecting the TMJ or the masticatory musculature."[1]

Verification and/or Correction of Midline Position

"Verification and/or correction of midline position describes an effort to ascertain and maintain the appropriate lateral position of the mandible in its forward position, often similar in lateral dimensions to the nonprotruded (nontreatment) position."[1]

Verification and/or Correction of Occlusion

"Verification and/or correction of occlusion describes an effort to ascertain balanced occlusal forces on the oral appliance both bilaterally and anteriorly-posteriorly. This balance may be altered as the mandible is advanced or as muscles alternatively relax or contract with use. This may encompass consideration of changes to the vertical dimension of the oral appliance."[1]

Habitual Occlusion

"Habitual occlusion refers to the position of closure between the dental arches in which the patient feels the teeth fit most comfortably with minimal feeling of stress in the muscles and joints."[1]

"Note: the term "habitual occlusion" refers to the patient's most comfortable position of jaw closure at any specific time. Many terms have been used to describe the interarch relationship of the maxilla and mandible, often with the intent of providing a reproducible position for restorative purposes. Terms such as centric relation, centric occlusion, maximum intercuspation, bite of convenience, and intercuspation position have also been used. This article favors the term 'habitual occlusion' because as many as 85% of the patients using OAT for more than 5 years demonstrate altered occlusal relationships from baseline."[1,2]

Isometric and Passive Jaw-Stretching Exercises

"Isometric and passive jaw-stretching exercises include instructing patients to move the mandible against resistance both vertically and laterally and to stretch the mandibular range of motion assisted by the fingers, targeting the masticatory muscles. Examples include instructing a patient to move the mandible against gentle resistance both vertically and laterally within their physiologic range of motion and using finger pressure to stretch the lateral pterygoid, temporalis, and master muscles. These have been shown to decrease the level of discomfort and improve adherence to OAT.[3] Duration and frequency of exercises will be dependent on the ease with which the patient is able to reestablish occlusion."[1]

Conservative Titration

"Conservative titration refers to the minimal amount of advancement of the appliance required to manage sleep disordered breathing. Aarab and colleagues[4] demonstrated that the number of side effects increases as protrusion exceeds 50% from baseline. Moreover, research reveals that 50% and 75% protrusion can be equally effective in groups of patients with mild to moderate OSA."[1,5]

SIDE-EFFECT RECOMMENDATIONS
Here Follows the Specific Recommendations of the Consensus Panel Followed by Some Key Bulleted Points for Each

Section 1: temporomandibular joint–related side effects
Care must be taken to differentiate the various different terms used to describe problems with the TMJ and associated musculature by the various different groups of practitioners involved in this field. It is also important to note here that myofascial pain and TMJ degeneration were not discovered in the research evaluated on this topic and were not included as specific side effects under consideration for this reason.

Transient morning jaw pain "Watchful waiting, palliative care, isometric contraction and passive jaw exercise, and decreasing the titration rate are considered first line of treatment to manage transient jaw pain."[1]

- This discomfort is considered mild and transient during the day following the use of OAT
- Usually originating from the muscles of mastication, this is unlikely to cause OAT abandonment
- Conservative titration should be adhered to
- Active surveillance is indicated to rule out pain originating from the joint(s)
- Reassurance, muscle massage, application of heat, and relaxation techniques are suggested[6,7]
- Isometric contraction and jaw exercises have been shown to be effective in relieving muscle discomfort[7]
- Decreasing titration rate may help alleviate symptoms[4]
- If symptoms continue, worsen during the day, last more than a few weeks, or interfere with normal function they should be considered *persistent* (see the next section)

Persistent temporomandibular joint pain " Palliative care, isometric contraction, and passive jaw-stretching exercises, verifying or correcting midline positions, appliance adjustment, decreasing the titration rate, decreasing advancement, and conducting a temporomandibular disorder (TMD) workup and management are considered first line of treatment to manage persistent TMJ pain. Placing posterior stops or anterior discluding elements, decreasing wearing time, and temporarily discontinuing use of OAT are considered second-line treatment. If these treatment options are insufficient or inappropriate, using a daytime intraoral orthotic, prescribing a steroid dose pack, recommending a different oral appliance (OA) design, referring to a dental specialist or additional health care provider, and permanently discontinuing OAT also may be appropriate."[1]

- Conservative titration should be adhered to (see common management techniques)
- Patients should be reassured that both TMJ baseline discomfort and discomfort associated with OA use is likely to decrease with time and continued use of the oral appliance[7–10]
- Proper documentation throughout resolution is important
- Rest, soft diet, and anti-inflammatory medications should be considered
- Isometric contraction and jaw exercises have been shown to be effective in relieving muscle discomfort[7]

- Decreasing the advancement rate may help speed relief of TMJ symptoms, but should be weighed against the decreasing therapeutic effect of the appliance
- In appliances in which there are both left and right advancement mechanisms, ensure that these advancements have been applied in even value
- As mentioned in the consensus paper, "refractory temporomandibular symptoms related to OAT are uncommon"[1]
- Consider an appliance that allows more jaw movement
- Consider placing posterior or anterior acrylic stops
- Decrease the time of appliance wear
- Limited steroid dose pack prescription where indicated
- If the previous items are ineffective or inapplicable, consider discontinuation of OAT; any decision to abandon OAT needs to be done in conjunction with the patient's physician to be sure that replacement therapy is planned

Tenderness in the muscles of mastication " Palliative care, watchful waiting, verifying or correcting midline positions, use of a morning occlusal guide, and isometric contraction and passive jaw-stretching exercises are considered first line of treatment to manage tenderness in the muscles of mastication. Decreasing OA advancement, vertical dimension, and the rate of forward titration; modifying the acrylic; and temporarily discontinuing use of OAT are considered second-line treatments. If these treatment options are insufficient or inappropriate, recommending a different OA design, referring to a dental specialist or additional health care provider, and permanently discontinuing OAT also may be appropriate. In very rare instances, increasing OA advancement may be indicated."[1]

- Muscle massage, application of heat (or ice if inflammation is present)
- Isometric and/or relaxation techniques[7]
- Balance left and right protrusive forces
- Morning occlusal guide
- Conservative titration should be adhered to
- Decrease the rate of titration or overall advancement position; care to balance against the decreasing therapeutic effect[4,11]
- Decrease vertical dimension of appliance
- Allow for more lateral movement of the mandible
- Temporarily discontinue OAT (then potentially restart in a more retruded position and advancing more slowly)

- Rarely, in some specific cases, advancement might achieve better resolution of OSA and quiet muscular activity
- Selective serotonin reuptake inhibitors also have the ability to affect changes on the tonicity of the muscles of mastication. These should be managed in conjunction with the treating physician if they are interfering with the patient's ability to tolerate treatment
- Consider referral to additional medical specialist, including a physical therapist, or a dentist with advanced training in TMD
- If the previous items are ineffective or inapplicable, consider discontinuation of OAT; any decision to abandon OAT needs to be done in conjunction with the patient's physician to be sure that replacement therapy is planned

Joint sounds "Watchful waiting is considered first line of treatment to manage joint sounds caused as a result of using OAs. If these treatment options are insufficient or inappropriate, temporary or permanent discontinuation of the OAT can also be considered as a treatment option."[1]

- These side effects are usually transient and resolve with time
- If these sounds coincide with persistent pain, it may be necessary to abandon OAT; as usual, the practitioner must be certain alternative therapy is planned
- Conservative titration should be adhered to

Section 2: intraoral tissue–related side effects
Soft tissue and tongue irritation "Palliative care and appliance modification are considered first line of treatment to manage soft tissue and tongue irritation side effects. Temporarily discontinuing use of the OA is considered a second-line treatment. If these treatment options are insufficient or inappropriate, orthodontic wax and switching to a different OA design also may be considered appropriate."[1]

- These are most commonly due to mechanical trauma
- Topical agents and/or appliance modifications are suggested
- Consider a switch to different OA design
- If the preceding items are ineffective or inapplicable, consider discontinuation of OAT; any decision to abandon OAT needs to be done in conjunction with the patient's physician to be sure that replacement therapy is planned

Gingival irritation "Modification of the appliance and palliative care are considered first-line treatment to manage gingival irritation. Discontinuing use of OAT temporarily is considered second-line treatment."[1]

- Appliance modifications
- Commonly due to mechanical trauma
- If the previous items are ineffective or inapplicable, consider discontinuation of OAT; any decision to abandon OAT needs to be done in conjunction with the patient's physician to be sure that replacement therapy is planned.

Excessive salivation "Watchful waiting is considered first line of treatment to manage excessive salivation/drooling. Modification to the appliance is considered second-line treatment. If these treatment options are insufficient or inappropriate, prescribing medications to decrease salivary input also may be appropriate."[1]

- Modification to the appliance should be considered after a period of watchful waiting, as this is normal and expectable for the first few weeks.
- This may include, but is not limited to decreasing vertical dimension to allow for better lip seal with the appliance in place.
- Mouth shields and oral obturators can be added to the appliance to help with the oral seal.

Dry mouth "Palliative care, watchful waiting, and decreasing vertical dimension of the device to encourage lip seal, are considered first line of treatment to manage dry mouth. Modification of the appliance and techniques for discouraging mouth breathing are considered second-line treatment. If these treatment options are insufficient or inappropriate, avoiding commercial mouth rinses with alcohol or peroxide, mouth-taping, and referring to an additional health care provider may also be considered appropriate."[1]

- Decreasing the vertical dimension can improve lip seal and discourage mouth breathing
- Ensure adequate hydration
- Limit over-the-counter substances that contribute to dry mouth
- Check with the physician to evaluate prescriptions that might cause xerostomia
- Consult with the otolaryngologist if nasal patency is problematic

Section 3: occlusal changes
Altered occlusal contacts/bite changes "Watchful waiting, jaw-stretching exercises, and use of a morning occlusal guide are considered first line of treatment to manage altered occlusal

contacts or bite changes. Chewing hard gum in the mornings and making modifications to the appliance are considered second-line treatment. If these treatment options are insufficient or inappropriate, discontinuing OAT temporarily or permanently may also be appropriate."[1]

- Adhere to conservative titration: greater titration increases the magnitude of force that in turn increases potential side effects[4,12,13]
- Posterior open bites occur commonly[7,14–19]
- Patients easily tolerate these changes and commonly are unaware of them[4,7,16,20,21]
- Morning occlusal guides are recommended
- Jaw-stretching exercises to help reseat the condyle and relieve muscle stiffness[22]
- Modify ill-fitting appliance
- If the previous items are ineffective or inapplicable, consider discontinuation of OAT; any decision to abandon OAT needs to be done in conjunction with the patient's physician to be sure that replacement therapy is planned
- Inform patient of change, continue with "watchful waiting"

Incisor changes "Watchful waiting, use of a morning occlusal guide. and modification to the appliance are considered first line of treatment to manage incisor angulation and position changes. If these treatment options are insufficient or inappropriate, recommending a different OA design and discontinuing OAT permanently may also be appropriate treatment options."[1]

- Anterior crossbites occur in 62% of all patients after 11 years[23] (at least 1, but commonly 4 teeth)
- Some tooth movements are not detrimental and could be considered beneficial
- Inform patient of change, continue with "watchful waiting"
- Relieve acrylic if necessary
- Proper documentation is important, the use of serial casts and measurements is advised
- Use of a morning occlusal guide is recommended

Decreased overjet and overbite "Watchful waiting, isometric contraction and passive jaw-stretching exercises, and use of a morning occlusal guide are considered first line of treatment to manage decreased overjet and overbite. Chewing hard gum in the morning is considered a second-line treatment."[1]

- More than 85% of all patients will experience some change[2]

- Some bite changes are not considered detrimental and may actually be considered beneficial
- Patients commonly are unaware of these changes
- Inform patient of change, continue with "watchful waiting"
- Morning occlusal guides are recommended
- Isometric passive jaw-stretching exercises to aid in reestablishing normal occlusion[22]

Alterations in positions of the mandibular canines and molars "Watchful waiting and use of a morning occlusal guide are considered first line of treatment to manage altered positions of mandibular canines and molars."[1]

- Mesial shift of mandibular canines and molars have been noted in as many as 27% of patients after just a few years[11,17,24]
- Multiple clinical evaluations during the first year of use
- Regular follow-up at yearly intervals[25]
- Inform patient of change, continue with "watchful waiting"
- Some tooth movements are not detrimental and could be considered beneficial
- Morning occlusal guides may help reestablish pretreatment occlusion

Interproximal gaps "Watchful waiting, use of a morning occlusal guide, adjusting ball clasps, and making modifications to the appliance are considered first line of treatment to manage interproximal gaps. If these treatment options are insufficient or inappropriate, use of a distal wraparound retainer and restoration of contact areas may be appropriate."[1]

- Common occurrence, especially in the mandible of patients with angle class I[2,26]
- Can lead to decay and or periodontal disease if not corrected
- Morning occlusal guide recommended
- Inform patient of change, continue with "watchful waiting"
- Reduction of the interproximal acrylic, removal of ball clasps, and/or addition of material in careful application to specific areas may be considered
- Distal wraparound spring may be considered

Section 4: damage to teeth or restorations
Tooth mobility "Palliative care and modifying the appliance are considered first line of treatment to manage tooth mobility. Decreasing the titration rate is considered second-line treatment. If these treatment options are insufficient or inappropriate,

daytime/fixed splinting of teeth also may be appropriate."[1]

- Palliative care where necessary
- Modification of the appliance if applicable
- Decrease the titration rate
- Daytime or fixed splinting of the teeth
- Consider a switch to different OA design
- If the previous items are ineffective or inapplicable, consider discontinuation of OAT; any decision to abandon OAT needs to be done in conjunction with the patient's physician to be sure that replacement therapy is planned

Tooth fractures or damage to dental restorations "Modifying the appliance and referral to a general/restorative dentist are considered first line of treatment to manage tooth fractures or damage to dental restorations. If these treatment options are insufficient or inappropriate, recommending a different OA design also may be appropriate."[1]

- Modify the appliance where appropriate
- Refer to the primary care dentist where necessary
- Consider a switch to different OA design

Section 5: appliance issues
Appliance breakage "Repairing or replacing the appliance is considered first line of treatment to manage appliance breakage. If these treatment options are insufficient or inappropriate, recommending a different OA design also may be appropriate."[1]

- A 2-year study demonstrated a 60% breakage rate with 40% of patients needing a new appliance[21]
- Frequent fracture of acrylic, particularly in patients with bruxism
- Breakage commonly in the telescoping mechanism of a Herbst appliance[27]

Allergies to appliance materials "Removing the allergenic material and temporary discontinuation of OA use are considered first line of treatment to manage allergies to appliance material. If these treatment options are insufficient or inappropriate, referring to another health care provider also may be considered as a treatment option."[1]

- Under cured methyl methacrylate, acrylic can more likely cause reaction by leaking monomer via porosity of the appliance
- Pressure and heat curing of methyl methacrylate may decrease sensitivity reaction
- Nickel, a common allergen, is a common component of stainless steel hardware

Gagging "Modifications to the appliance are considered first line of treatment to manage gagging. Deprogramming the gag reflex is considered second-line treatment. If these treatment options are insufficient or inappropriate, recommendation of a different OA design also may be appropriate."[1]

- Allow for freedom of movement, especially uninhibited opening and lateral movement
- Consider thinner, less bulky appliances with more tongue space to facilitate swallowing
- Cognitive behavioral therapy/desensitizing techniques may help

Anxiety "Watchful waiting and use of desensitization techniques are considered first line of treatment to manage anxiety. If these treatment options are insufficient or inappropriate, recommending a different OA design and referring to a different health care provider also may be appropriate."[1]

- Wear the appliance for some time before bedtime for desensitization
- Choose appliances that allow for free lateral and vertical movement
- Choose appliances with less bulk

Additional concerns There remains one additional serious negative "effect" of OAT that warrants discussion here. Although not a side effect per se, this negative effect could very well be the most significant unintended consequence of OAT, and the most threatening to our patients' well-being. The sheer bulk of the OA as it is introduced into an already crowded oral environment has the potential to increase the apnea pressure, at least until forward posture through titration can compensate. This does not necessarily need to be accompanied by any worsening overt signs or symptoms. Although likely to help substantially, by no means is OAT a guarantee for improvement of OSA; not all patients in the available research studies demonstrate positive effect. Finding atypical responders is not infrequent and should caution all practitioners' activity. There also exist a certain number of patients who worsen past a certain point of titration, thus missing what is commonly referred to as the "sweet spot" of maximum efficacy. As has been stated many times, adherence to conservative titration is important.

It is critical to make sure that proper follow-up with a physician is encouraged for the objective measure of the presence, absence, and severity of residual apnea. The diagnosis of this disease belongs in the hands of those legally licensed and responsible for it. Without this objective analysis, we may have not only failed to help alleviate disease, but could have actually introduced more harm than had we not intervened. Keep in mind that Home Sleep Apnea Testing is not nearly as predictable as a full polysomnography, especially in mild and moderate OSA. The American Dental Association Principles of Ethics and Code of Professional Conduct insists on 3 important factors: veracity, nonmaleficence, and beneficence. The principle of veracity implies that objective measures of OAT titration success need to be accurate in all the ranges of OSA. The remaining 2 factors insist that in an attempt to help a patient we take care to do no harm.

SUMMARY

As previously mentioned, there is a serious need to consider all potential side effects thoughtfully before commencing individual treatment. Although many of these side effects are self-limiting, easily corrected, or innocuous, others are difficult or impossible to correct and can affect the patient in some serious ways. If alternative treatment is not acceptable, the carefully weighed risk of no therapy is what allows practitioners to justify these likely problems to coexist with OAT. As this field evolves, new information is discovered and new products are introduced at a rather rapid pace, continuing education and prudent practice is critical to ethical care in the practice of DSM.

REFERENCES

1. Sheats RD, Schell TG, Blanton AO, et al. Management of side effects of oral appliance therapy for sleep disordered breathing. J Dent Sleep Med 2017;04(04):111–25.
2. Almeida FR, Lowe AA, Otsuka R, et al. Long-term sequelae of oral appliance therapy in obstructive sleep apnea patients: part 2. Study-model analysis. Am J Orthod Dentofacial Orthop 2006;129(2):205–13.
3. Cunali PA, Almeida FR, Santos CD, et al. Mandibular exercises improve mandibular advancement device therapy for obstructive sleep apnea. Sleep Breath 2011;15(4):717–27.
4. Aarab G, Lobbezoo F, Hamburger HL, et al. Effects of an oral appliance with different mandibular protrusion positions at a constant vertical dimension on obstructive sleep apnea. Clin Oral Investig 2010; 14(3):339–45.
5. Tegelberg A, Walker-Engstrom ML, Vestling O, et al. Two different degrees of mandibular advancement with a dental appliance in treatment of patients with mild to moderate obstructive sleep apnea. Acta Odontol Scand 2003;61(6):356–62.

6. Chen H, Lowe AA. Updates in oral appliance therapy for snoring and obstructive sleep apnea. Sleep Breath 2013;17(2):473–86.

7. Perez CV, de Leeuw R, Okeson JP, et al. The incidence and prevalence of temporomandibular disorders and posterior open bite in patients receiving mandibular advancement device therapy for obstructive sleep apnea. Sleep Breath 2013;17(1): 323–32.

8. Cohen-Levy J, Garcia R, Petelle B, et al. Treatment of the obstructive sleep apnea syndrome in adults by mandibular advancement device: the state of the art. Int Orthod 2009;7(3):287–304.

9. Fransson AM, Tegelberg A, Leissner L, et al. Effects of a mandibular protruding device on the sleep of patients with obstructive sleep apnea and snoring problems: a 2-year followup. Sleep Breath 2003; 7(3):131–41.

10. Doff MH, Veldhuis SK, Hoekema A, et al. Long-term oral appliance therapy in obstructive sleep apnea syndrome: a controlled study on temporomandibular side effects. Clin Oral Investig 2012;16(3):689–97.

11. Chen H, Lowe AA, de Almeida FR, et al. Three-dimensional computer-assisted study model analysis of long-term oral-appliance wear. Part 2. Side effects of oral appliances in obstructive sleep apnea patients. Am J Orthod Dentofacial Orthop 2008; 134(3):408–17.

12. Cohen-Levy J, Petelle B, Pinguet J, et al. Forces created by mandibular advancement devices in OSAS patients: a pilot study during sleep. Sleep Breath 2013;17(2):781–9.

13. Tegelberg A, Wilhelmsson B, Walker-Engstrom ML, et al. Effects and adverse events of a dental appliance for treatment of obstructive sleep apnoea. Swed Dent J 1999;23(4):117–26.

14. Vezina JP, Blumen MB, Buchet I, et al. Does propulsion mechanism influence the long-term side effects of oral appliances in the treatment of sleep-disordered breathing? Chest 2011;140(5):1184–91.

15. Rose EC, Schnegelsberg C, Staats R, et al. Occlusal side effects caused by a mandibular advancement appliance in patients with obstructive sleep apnea. Angle Orthod 2001;71(6):452–60.

16. Rose EC, Staats R, Virchow C Jr, et al. Occlusal and skeletal effects of an oral appliance in the treatment of obstructive sleep apnea. Chest 2002;122(3): 871–7.

17. Ueda H, Almeida FR, Lowe AA, et al. Changes in occlusal contact area during oral appliance therapy assessed on study models. Angle Orthod 2008; 78(5):866–72.

18. Marklund M, Legrell PE. An orthodontic oral appliance. Angle Orthod 2010;80(6):1116–21.

19. Doff MH, Hoekema A, Wijkstra PJ, et al. Oral appliance versus continuous positive airway pressure in obstructive sleep apnea syndrome: a 2-year follow-up. Sleep 2013;36(9):1289–96.

20. Marklund M, Sahlin C, Stenlund H, et al. Mandibular advancement device in patients with obstructive sleep apnea: long-term effects on apnea and sleep. Chest 2001;120(1):162–9.

21. Battagel JM, Kotecha B. Dental side-effects of mandibular advancement splint wear in patients who snore. Clin Otolaryngol 2005;30(2):149–56.

22. Ueda H, Almeida FR, Chen H, et al. Effect of 2 jaw exercises on occlusal function in patients with obstructive sleep apnea during oral appliance therapy: a randomized controlled trial. Am J Orthod Dentofacial Orthop 2009;135(4):430.e1–7 [discussion: 430–31].

23. Pliska BT, Nam H, Chen H, et al. Obstructive sleep apnea and mandibular advancement splints: occlusal effects and progression of changes associated with a decade of treatment. J Clin Sleep Med 2014;10(12):1285–91.

24. Almeida FR, Lowe AA, Sung JO, et al. Long-term sequelae of oral appliance therapy in obstructive sleep apnea patients: part 1. Cephalometric analysis. Am J Orthod Dentofacial Orthop 2006;129(2): 195–204.

25. AADSM treatment protocol: oral appliance therapy for sleep disordered breathing: an update for 2013. American Academy of Dental Sleep Medicine Web site; 2013. Available at: https://aadsm.org/docs/JDSM.04.04.pdf. Accessed August 23, 2017.

26. Doff MH, Finnema KJ, Hoekema A, et al. Long-term oral appliance therapy in obstructive sleep apnea syndrome: a controlled study on dental side effects. Clin Oral Investig 2013;17(2):475–82.

27. Martinez-Gomis J, Willaert E, Nogues L, et al. Five years of sleep apnea treatment with a mandibular advancement device. Side effects and technical complications. Angle Orthod 2010;80(1):30–6.

Oral Appliance Therapy and Temporomandibular Disorders

Noshir R. Mehta, BDS, DMD, MS,
Leopoldo P. Correa, BDS, MS*

KEYWORDS

- Oral appliance therapy • Temporomandibular disorders • Dental sleep medicine
- Mandibular advancement devices • Obstructive sleep apnea

KEY POINTS

- Temporomandibular disorders is an umbrella term for pain in the face, head, and neck.
- Cervical disorders are integral part of temporomandibular disorders.
- Three-dimensional maxillomandibular relationships are important in the assessment and management of temporomandibular disorders using appliance therapy.
- Sleep disorders and temporomandibular disorders are intimately related.
- Mandibular advancement devices (MADs) may have side effects on the temporomandibular disorders.

INTRODUCTION

Dental sleep medicine has evolved rapidly during the last few years thanks to the advancement in research related to the use and efficacy of oral appliance therapy. Oral appliances assist in holding the jaw forward during sleep to prevent the collapsibility of upper airway muscles; based on this function oral appliances are named mandibular advancement devices (MADs). However, the resultant advancement of the lower jaw in some patients may produce discomfort or pain in the masticatory muscles, temporomandibular joint (TMJ), and head and neck areas. This article presents a brief historical introduction of the field of sleep and focuses primarily on an overview of temporomandibular disorders (TMD), including clinical examination and management of common TMD symptoms developing from the use of MAD for obstructive sleep apnea (OSA).

Somnology has been of interest to many cultures throughout history. Mention of sleep has been found in Greek mythology where sleep was considered the transition between sleep and dead personified by the twin brothers Hypnos and Thanatos.[1] Sigmund Freud introduced the theory of the unconscious and dream interpretation; such theories influenced the surrealism style seen in the work of the Spanish painter Salvador Dali.[2,3]

Several theories of why we sleep have been described, including the adaptive-evolutionary, energy conservation, and the restorative theory, which has been the one that fulfills the most recent discoveries in the science of sleep medicine demonstrating that many of the major restorative functions in the body, such as muscle growth, tissue repair, protein synthesis, and growth hormone release, occur during sleep.[4]

Initial experiments leading toward the understanding of modern human sleep date back from

Tufts University School of Dental Medicine, 1 Kneeland Street, Boston, MA 0111, USA
* Corresponding author.
E-mail address: Leopoldo.correa@tufts.edu

Sleep Med Clin 13 (2018) 513–519
https://doi.org/10.1016/j.jsmc.2018.08.001
1556-407X/18/© 2018 Elsevier Inc. All rights reserved.

sleep.theclinics.com

1875 when the physician Richard Caton performed the first recording of brain electrical activity in animals and reported electrical properties of exposed cerebral hemispheres of rabbits and monkeys to the British Medical Association in Edinburgh. Similar work was done by Adolf Beck in Poland studying electrical brain activity of animals.[5] Hans Berger, a German psychiatrist, performed the first recording of brain activity in wakeful humans and discovered alpha waves assessed by what is still known today as the electroencephalogram.[6]

The first continuous overnight electroencephalogram recording in humans is attributed to Loomis and Harvey on tracings on miles of paper using an 8-ft-long drum polygraph.[7]

A landmark discovery in the measurement of sleep is attributed to Aserinsky and Kleitman[8] where, in 1953, they identified associated respiratory and cardiac effects during their sleep laboratory observations and later incorporated these findings into the stages of rapid eye movement sleep. The classification of rapid eye movement and non–rapid eye movement sleep cycles was proposed just few years later by Dement and Kleitman.[9]

Somnology and sleep medicine has expanded at an accelerated pace and has demonstrated evidence about metabolic consequences of sleep and sleep loss including the regulation of glucose metabolism, appetite, hormonal release, and cardiovascular function.[10,11] Acute periods of experimental sleep restriction have been shown to produce increased blood pressure, heightened sympathetic nervous system activity, and elevated levels of inflammatory markers.[12–14] The effect of sleep loss and sleep disorders has been shown to cause an important impact on public health, transportation safety, and industrial and engineering disasters.[15–17]

OSA is a common sleep disorder characterized by repetitive episodes of upper airway obstruction with efforts to breathe, resulting in reduction of blood oxygen saturation and ending with sleep arousal.[18] The pathophysiology, prevalence, risk factors, and health consequences have been reported extensively elsewhere.[19–24]

MADs have been proven to be effective in the management of OSA resulting in improvement of medical comorbidities as reported in an updated review by Sutherland and colleagues.[25] Clinical practice guidelines recommend the use of MAD by qualified dentists with knowledge in sleep medicine and with enough clinical competence in the management of common side effects including TMD symptoms.[26] The term "qualified dentist" is a designation provided by the American Academy of Dental Sleep Medicine, which is the leading professional association in this field. The term identifies dental professionals who have obtained the minimal educational requirements in dental sleep medicine from nonprofit organizations or accredited dental schools.

MANDIBULAR ADVANCEMENT DEVICES AND TEMPOROMANDIBULAR DISORDERS

MADs function by repositioning the lower jaw forward during sleep, which assists the advancement of the tongue and surrounding tissues with the goal to increase upper airway size and prevent collapsibility. In some patients, there may be a dose-dependent effect of mandibular advancement on oxygen saturation and pharyngeal mechanics as demonstrated by Kato and colleagues.[27] The TMJ must perform rotation and translation movements with the use of MADs; therefore. there is a potential risk of developing symptoms during the titration (advancement) of these devices. De Almeida and colleagues[28] reported the effect of mandibular posture at different increments on reduction of OSA severity and the morphologic assessment of condylar position in patients with MAD therapy. Their study demonstrated that reduction of OSA severity (measured by apnea-hypopnea index) was related to the dose-dependent effect on the amount of mandibular protrusion and at a 1-year follow-up MAD therapy proved to be innocuous for TMJ. In addition to the TMJ, the masticatory muscles may be affected and patients may complain about face pain. A study performed by Fransson and colleagues[29] assessed adverse events in the masticatory system after treatment with MADs during a 2-year follow-up. Patients reported high compliance rate of MAD use and no pain on jaw opening and side-side movement; some reported tiredness on jaw function, and others reported decrease in headaches ($P<.01$). Minor alterations in occlusion were reported.

TEMPOROMANDIBULAR JOINT–RELATED SIDE EFFECTS

Transient morning jaw pain is the most common pain related to wearing of oral appliances and seems to come from the mandible being held in an overnight position that is not comfortable. This tightness and pain is usually related to too much anterior positioning of the mandible leading to strain in the TMJs bilaterally. In cases where there is unilateral pain in the side of the face, this is usually related to muscular or myofascial pain and generally is treated by midlining the mandible and balancing the left and right sides on the intraoral appliance.[30,31] In cases where the vertical dimension is opened too far because of the thickness of the appliances being used, the main complaint is stiffness and tightness and pain in the back of the head and neck.[31,32] These are generally transient and quickly dissipate. The symptoms return if the thickness of the sleep device is not reduced.

Persistent TMJ pain may manifest if there is increase in pressure on the joints or if there is inflammation present in the joint spaces. Tenderness in the muscles of mastication is related to biting pressure on the posterior aspects of the appliance and/or an imbalance in the occlusal aspects of the appliance. TMJ sounds, such as clicking and popping, are usually improved by appliance therapy but may worsen in some patients.[30] Tooth injury caused by bruxism and soft tissue lacerations can happen if the oral appliance is not smooth and well balanced. Headaches and neck pain are a consequence of excessive vertical height of the appliance.

The Tufts Discomfort Scale developed by Mehta is used on every visit to monitor changes on symptoms related to 12 body sites. The Tufts Discomfort scale is a numeric scale based on a 1 to 10 scale. The scale is for left and right sides and is filled out by the patient each time they come in for a visit. The scale was first developed for research purposes, because by placing each one side by side the treatment specialist can track pain by day and by visit. In addition, the scale also looks at specific sites of pain and there is also a total score if needed. Mostly, the score tracks the effectiveness of treatment over time and allows one to see which symptom site is affected the most by whatever treatment is done. It also allows the patient to see the effectiveness of the treatment by their own responses and allows the doctor to have documentation on the same (**Fig. 1**).

MAXILLOMANDIBULAR EXAMINATION

Anatomic factors, such as structural abnormalities in the hard and soft tissues of maxillofacial area, may lead to an increased risk of upper airway compromise. Maxillomandibular harmony is a product of many structural considerations and physiologic processes. To achieve a stable maxillomandibular relationship, there must be a confluence of balanced muscle action, proper TMJ position, and distributed guiding contacts of teeth in the closing stroke. Maxillomandibular imbalance seems to have a direct relationship with the masticatory musculature.[33] Imbalances in the masticatory musculature may affect the postural muscles

of the head and neck and possibly the upper airway.[34] Mehta[34] described the "occlusal fencing concept" whereby the maxilla acts as a "fence" for the mandibular teeth. If the maxilla is constricted, then the mandibular teeth crowd to accommodate to the space allowed by the maxillary teeth, creating a retrusive position of the lower jaw and increasing the risk for the narrowing of the upper airway (**Fig. 2**).

CLINICAL EXAMINATION

Assessment of the head, face, and neck structures is essential in deciding on the appropriateness of MAD use. Preventing possible side effects requires an understanding of the three-dimensional mandibular position as it relates to the masticatory muscles, the TMJ, and head posture in sleep. The concept of the maxilla forming the boundary or "fence" for the mandible to function during day remains the same for at night. The difference is the upright head position versus lying down with the effect of gravity defining the position. In addition, the mandible tends to drift in sleep as the muscle tone decreases with a tendency to move posteriorly in the fence created by the maxilla (first occlusal fence) (**Fig. 3**). This then causes a distal movement of the tongue into the back of the throat further reducing the airway space (**Fig. 4**).

This dropping back of the mandible and subsequent reduction of the airway by the tongue then creates a possible "equal and opposite reaction" by the body as a defense mechanism. There is some evidence that this reaction may lead to the mandible being braced forward by the muscles of the jaw and neck to maintain the airway. This is suggested by the fact that most tooth wear seems to be in the lower anterior teeth, which one can see by having the patient bring the mandible forward to the point where the upper and lower teeth wear facets are matched to each other. At the start of the examination one must look at the frenal buccal midlines of the mandible (second occlusal fence) to the maxilla in its seated centric maximum intercuspal position (**Fig. 5**). If the mandibular frenum midline is more than 2 mm to one side of the maxillary midline frenum one must further investigate the possibility that bringing the mandible straight forward would adversely affect the TMJ unilaterally. The side to which the mandibular frenum is deviated generally tends to be the joint that is most affected and may act up when the MAD is worn overnight. Vertical dimension which is affected by the thickness of the MAD worn and its effect on the airway and the muscle of the head and neck is the third occlusal dimension significantly affecting the neck. (**Fig. 6**).

Patient Name:_____   Date:_____

For each part of the body there are two horizontal rows, one for the left and one for the right. Please report the average discomfort over the last two weeks by circling a rating from "0" to "10" which best reflects your discomfort. If you have discomfort on both sides, circle both rows.

	SIDE	NONE										SEVERE
Bite Symptoms or Bite Changes	Left	0	1	2	3	4	5	6	7	8	9	10
	Right	0	1	2	3	4	5	6	7	8	9	10
TMJ pain	Left	0	1	2	3	4	5	6	7	8	9	10
	Right	0	1	2	3	4	5	6	7	8	9	10
TMJ sounds	Left	0	1	2	3	4	5	6	7	8	9	10
	Right	0	1	2	3	4	5	6	7	8	9	10
Headaches	Left	0	1	2	3	4	5	6	7	8	9	10
	Right	0	1	2	3	4	5	6	7	8	9	10
Facial Pain	Left	0	1	2	3	4	5	6	7	8	9	10
	Right	0	1	2	3	4	5	6	7	8	9	10
Eye Symptoms	Left	0	1	2	3	4	5	6	7	8	9	10
	Right	0	1	2	3	4	5	6	7	8	9	10
Ear Pain	Left	0	1	2	3	4	5	6	7	8	9	10
	Right	0	1	2	3	4	5	6	7	8	9	10
Stuffy Ear or Ringing Sounds	Left	0	1	2	3	4	5	6	7	8	9	10
	Right	0	1	2	3	4	5	6	7	8	9	10
Neck Pain	Left	0	1	2	3	4	5	6	7	8	9	10
	Right	0	1	2	3	4	5	6	7	8	9	10
Arm/Hand/Finger Numbness, tingling or pain	Left	0	1	2	3	4	5	6	7	8	9	10
	Right	0	1	2	3	4	5	6	7	8	9	10
Upper Back Pain	Left	0	1	2	3	4	5	6	7	8	9	10
	Right	0	1	2	3	4	5	6	7	8	9	10
Lower back Pain	Left	0	1	2	3	4	5	6	7	8	9	10
	Right	0	1	2	3	4	5	6	7	8	9	10
Overall Pain Score:		0	1	2	3	4	5	6	7	8	9	10

COMMENTS:

Patient's Signature:_____

Fig. 1. Tufts discomfort scale.

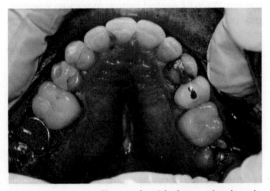

Fig. 2. Narrow maxillary arch with deep palatal vault.

NEED FOR HEAD, NECK, AND MASTICATORY MUSCLES EXAMINATION

In addition to the masseter, temporalis, lateral, and medial pterygoid muscles it is well known that the head and neck muscles participate in the act of chewing and swallowing. Furthermore, electromyogram studies have also shown that the anterior and posterior neck muscles interact in maintaining head posture, which affects jaw position.[35] For the lower jaw to close forcefully enough to cut through and chew through the food it requires that force be created between the teeth. The head needs to be stabilized so the maxilla acts as the "ceiling" against which the lower arch can push against to masticate the food. The

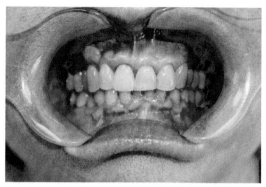

Fig. 3. Mouth closed in maximum interincisal position. Note the posterior displacement of the mandible to allow the lower teeth to fit into the confines of the upper arch.

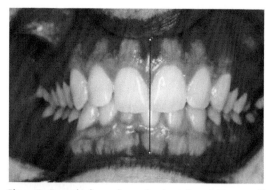

Fig. 5. Frenal buccal and dental midlines off alignment.

neck muscles are the stabilizers of the head against the mandible's force.

Head and neck muscles and the cervical spine are also important in maintaining airway during sleep and awake periods. During sleep periods the head and jaw posture changes as individuals sleep or their sides, prone, or supine. The mandible then shifts and when the airway is adversely affected by mandibular displacement posteriorly or the tongue drops back into the airway there is a possibility that stenting by the submental muscles brings the anterior teeth into contact to hold the airway space open in sleep. This may be the reason the lower anterior teeth usually show the most wear in sleep patients who parafunction.[36] The examiner must palpate all the head and neck muscle groups for tenderness to palpation and for tightness and pain.

TEMPOROMANDIBULAR JOINT

Palpation and examination of the range of motion of the TMJ is essential because the most common

side effect of mandibular advancement using MADs is joint pain and may be accompanied with joint noises, such as clicking or popping. Midline shifts of the mandible evidenced by examining midline frenal positions in centric occlusion can help preventatively assess the potential for such problems. The TMJ contralateral to the mandibular frenal deviation is the side that the patient feels being too far forward when the bite registration recording is made. Treatment of this issue requires that the mandible be centered with the frenal midlines being no more than 1.25 mm off before bringing the mandible forward for the MAD position. In addition, a morning repositioner like the one designed by Correa (**Fig. 7**) is used for bringing the mandible back to its normal position. The patient wears the device for about 15 minutes after removal of sleep oral device.

SUMMARY

There have been many concepts proposed for the evaluation of dental occlusion. These concepts mostly have been dentally static positions, designed for bilateral balance with forces vertically

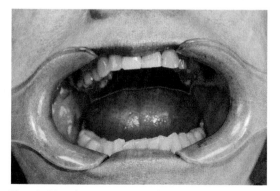

Fig. 4. Mouth open. Note drape position of the tongue over the lower posterior teeth.

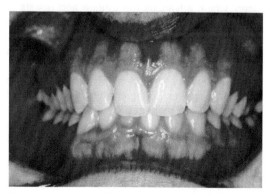

Fig. 6. Lingual position of molars developing deep overbite/loss of vertical dimension of occlusion.

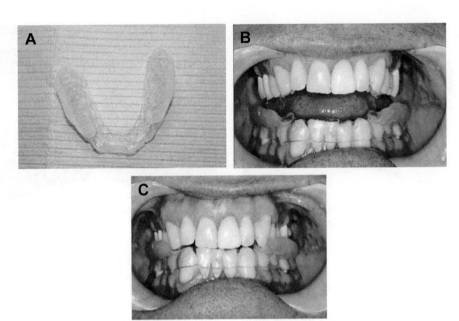

Fig. 7. (*A*) Correa Morning Aligner (CMA) design. (*B*) CMA in the mouth with occlusal grooves as occlusal guidance. (*C*) CMA with patient in full closure.

aligned on the teeth. Occlusion should be considered not only as a static concept but also as a dynamic one that can affect the craniofacial and cervical systems. For a stable dental occlusion, there must be a confluence of balanced muscle action, properly positioned TMJs, and distributed guiding contacts in the closing movement. Clinical examination is the tool to assist in determining a stable function between jaw position, muscle function, and TMJ stability, and it is recommended that bite registration techniques follow this three-dimensional assessment of dental occlusion to minimize TMD side effects with the use of MADs. This review described a simple and understandable approach for assessment and management of common TMD symptoms.

Oral appliances manage OSA function by repositioning the lower jaw in a forward position during sleep, which advances the tongue and results in improved upper airway patency. The forces created by these devices, their design features, and the extent of the therapeutic jaw protrusion may produce disharmony within the TMJs, neck, and masticatory muscles. These symptoms commonly appear during the first few weeks of therapy and are managed by making subtle adjustments to the appliances. Several studies have demonstrated occlusal side effects of these devices with long-term use.

Current clinical guidelines recommend that following diagnosis and referral from a physician, qualified dentists can use oral appliances among patients with mild to moderate OSA or in particular cases of severe sleep apnea in which patients are noncompliant with or unable to use positive airway pressure therapy. Clinical techniques, such as the use of morning jaw aligners like the one described in this review and the performance of jaw exercises, have been developed to minimize occlusal symptoms during oral appliance therapy; however, these approaches require further research to confirm their validity and long-term efficacy.

As dental sleep medicine continues to grow, it is essential that dentists who use oral appliances for OSA also understand the management of side effects, including occlusal symptoms, and adhere to current standards of dental sleep medicine practice.

REFERENCES

1. Bresson J, Liu N, Fischler M, et al. Anesthesia, sleep and death: from mythology to the operating room. Anesth Analg 2013;117(5):1257–9.
2. Parsons T. The interpretation of dreams by Sigmund Freud. Daedalus 1974;103:91–6.
3. Martinez-Conde S, Conley D, Hine H, et al. Marvels of illusion: illusion and perception in the art of Salvador Dali. Front Hum Neurosci 2015;9:496.
4. Siegel JM. Clues to the functions of mammalian sleep. Nature 2005;437(7063):1264–71.
5. Coenen A, Zayachkivska O. Adolf Beck: a pioneer in electroencephalography in between Richard Caton and Hans Berger. Adv Cogn Psychol 2013;9(4):216–21.

6. Schulte W. Hans Berger: a biography of the discoverer of the electroencephalogram. Munch Med Wochenschr 1959;101(22):977–80 [in German].

7. Davis H, Davis PA, Loomis AL, et al. Changes in human brain potentials during the onset of sleep. Science 1937;86(2237):448–50.

8. Aserinsky E, Kleitman N. Regularly occurring periods of eye motility, and concomitant phenomena, during sleep. Science 1953;118(3062):273–4.

9. Dement W, Kleitman N. Cyclic variations in EEG during sleep and their relation to eye movements, body motility, and dreaming. Electroencephalogr Clin Neurophysiol 1957;9(4):673–90.

10. Morselli L, Leproult R, Balbo M, et al. Role of sleep duration in the regulation of glucose metabolism and appetite. Best Pract Res Clin Endocrinol Metab 2010;24(5):687–702.

11. Van Cauter E, Spiegel K, Tasali E, et al. Metabolic consequences of sleep and sleep loss. Sleep Med 2008;9(Suppl 1):S23–8.

12. Meier-Ewert HK, Ridker PM, Rifai N, et al. Effect of sleep loss on C-reactive protein, an inflammatory marker of cardiovascular risk. J Am Coll Cardiol 2004;43(4):678–83.

13. Spiegel K, Leproult R, Van Cauter E. Impact of sleep debt on metabolic and endocrine function. Lancet 1999;354(9188):1435–9.

14. Tochikubo O, Ikeda A, Miyajima E, et al. Effects of insufficient sleep on blood pressure monitored by a new multibiomedical recorder. Hypertension 1996;27(6):1318–24.

15. Colten HR, Altevogt BM, editors. Sleep disorders and sleep deprivation: an unmet public health problem. Washington, DC: National Academies Press; 2006.

16. Roehrs T, Beare D, Zorick F, et al. Sleepiness and ethanol effects on simulated driving. Alcohol Clin Exp Res 1994;18(1):154–8.

17. Sanna A. Obstructive sleep apnoea, motor vehicle accidents, and work performance. Chron Respir Dis 2013;10(1):29–33.

18. Sleep-related breathing disorders in adults: recommendations for syndrome definition and measurement techniques in clinical research. The Report of an American Academy of Sleep Medicine Task Force. Sleep 1999;22(5):667–89.

19. Remmers JE, deGroot WJ, Sauerland EK, et al. Pathogenesis of upper airway occlusion during sleep. J Appl Physiol Respir Environ Exerc Physiol 1978; 44(6):931–8.

20. Tishler PV, Larkin EK, Schluchter MD, et al. Incidence of sleep-disordered breathing in an urban adult population: the relative importance of risk factors in the development of sleep-disordered breathing. JAMA 2003;289(17):2230–7.

21. Peppard PE, Young T, Barnet JH, et al. Increased prevalence of sleep-disordered breathing in adults. Am J Epidemiol 2013;177(9):1006–14.

22. Young T, Skatrud J, Peppard PE. Risk factors for obstructive sleep apnea in adults. JAMA 2004; 291(16):2013–6.

23. Yaggi HK, Concato J, Kernan WN, et al. Obstructive sleep apnea as a risk factor for stroke and death. N Engl J Med 2005;353(19):2034–41.

24. Peker Y, Carlson J, Hedner J. Increased incidence of coronary artery disease in sleep apnoea: a long-term follow-up. Eur Respir J 2006;28(3):596–602.

25. Sutherland K, Vanderveken OM, Tsuda H, et al. Oral appliance treatment for obstructive sleep apnea: an update. J Clin Sleep Med 2014;10(2):215–27.

26. Ramar K, Dort LC, Katz SG, et al. Clinical practice guideline for the treatment of obstructive sleep apnea and snoring with oral appliance therapy: an update for 2015. J Clin Sleep Med 2015;11(7):773–827.

27. Kato J, Isono S, Tanaka A, et al. Dose-dependent effects of mandibular advancement on pharyngeal mechanics and nocturnal oxygenation in patients with sleep-disordered breathing. Chest 2000; 117(4):1065–72.

28. de Almeida FR, Bittencourt LR, de Almeida CI, et al. Effects of mandibular posture on obstructive sleep apnea severity and the temporomandibular joint in patients fitted with an oral appliance. Sleep 2002; 25(5):507–13.

29. Fransson AM, Tegelberg A, Johansson A, et al. Influence on the masticatory system in treatment of obstructive sleep apnea and snoring with a mandibular protruding device: a 2-year follow-up. Am J Orthod Dentofacial Orthop 2004;126(6):687–93.

30. Mehta NR, Forgione AG, Rosenbaum RS, et al. "TMJ" triad of dysfunctions: a biologic basis of diagnosis and treatment. J Mass Dent Soc 1984;33(4): 173–6, 212–3.

31. Wongwatana S, Kronman JH, Clark RE, et al. Anatomic basis for disk displacement in temporomandibular joint (TMJ) dysfunction. Am J Orthod Dentofacial Orthop 1994;105(3):257–64.

32. Abduljabbar T, Mehta NR, Forgione AG, et al. Effect of increased maxillo-mandibular relationship on isometric strength in TMD patients with loss of vertical dimension of occlusion. Cranio 1997;15(1):57–67.

33. Fu AS, Mehta NR, Forgione AG, et al. Maxillomandibular relationship in TMD patients before and after short-term flat plane bite plate therapy. Cranio 2003; 21(3):172–9.

34. Mehta NR. Redefining dental occlusion. Cranio 2017;35(1):3.

35. Ceneviz C, Mehta NR, Forgione A, et al. The immediate effect of changing mandibular position on the EMG activity of the masseter, temporalis, sternocleidomastoid, and trapezius muscles. Cranio 2006; 24(4):237–44.

36. Mehta NR. Is there a commonality of occlusion for dental, TMD and obstructive sleep apnea patients? Thoughts on a snowy day. Cranio 2018;36(2):73.

Obstructive Sleep Apnea's Connections with Clinical Dentistry

Steve Carstensen, DDS[a,b,c,d,e,f],*

KEYWORDS

- Office systems • Disruption • Airway • Oral appliances • Team growth • Medical decision-making
- Treatment planning • Apnea

KEY POINTS

- Dentists trained to see airway-related problems will see the need to change office systems to incorporate this new knowledge. The disruption that results will require significant leadership skills.
- Getting to know their patients, completing a physical examination, and developing a treatment plan will all require a new and deeper relationship between every dental team member and the patient.
- Devoting time during team meetings with learning exercises will help in gaining comfort with why the new service can be fun, challenging, and rewarding as the team becomes comfortable with communication needs.

INTRODUCTION

There is nothing simple about planning dental restorative care. Dentists are responsible for considering every aspect of the person's health during the initial encounter in which the patient expects a thorough evaluation, assessment of condition, and recommendation by the doctor. As the relationship continues, new opportunities for health improvements may arise from changes to the patient's oral and general health, or as the dentist gains clinical knowledge through education and experience. Commonly, dentists are learning about sleep-related breathing disorders (SRBD). This article discusses the impact the presence of SRBDs can have on treatment planning, better labeled medical decision-making (MDM).

Every dental student learns the tools of examination and documentation of oral health and disease. If the only considerations were the health of teeth, periodontium, oral tissues, muscles of mastication and temporomandibular joints, then dental school and clinical practice prepare the dentist well for MDM limited to those areas. From the earliest days of modern dentistry, however, there have been visionaries such as Dr L.D. Pankey. Pankey and Davis[1] taught that there is much more to the patient than can be described so simply. Because nothing in the body is disconnected from any other part, dentists cannot take inventory of the plus and minus aspects of oral structures and make fully informed medical decisions. Acquiring a proper history and physical

Disclosure Statement: Advisory board, SleepArchiTx.

[a] Private Practice, Premier Sleep Associates, 636 120th Avenue NE A204, Bellevue, WA 98005, USA; [b] Medmark Media, LLC, Dental Sleep Practice Magazine, 15720 N. Greenway Hayden Loop, Suite 9, Scottsdale, AZ 85260, USA; [c] The Pankey Institute, One Crandon Boulevard Key Biscayne, FL 33149, USA; [d] Louisiana State University Health Continuing Dental Education, 1100 Florida Avenue, New Orleans, LA 70119, USA; [e] Department of Continuing Dental Education, The University of the Pacific, San Francisco, CA, USA; [f] Spear Education, 7201 E Princess Boulevard, Scottsdale, AZ 85255, USA

* 2908 181st Avenue Northeast, Redmond, WA 98052.

E-mail address: SeattleSleepEd@gmail.com

Sleep Med Clin 13 (2018) 521–529
https://doi.org/10.1016/j.jsmc.2018.07.004
1556-407X/18/© 2018 Elsevier Inc. All rights reserved.

examination (PE) makes appropriate MDM possible but the process challenges office systems and dental teams. After the data are assembled, the dentist merges health details, as well as the potential for any dental treatment, to affect the whole patient while tending to oral health needs that might be more obvious. At the same time, an SRBD may limit the choices the dentist can recommend, affect the prognosis of disease control, require collaboration with other medical providers, and shape expectations of ongoing disease management. The impact on a dental practice of taking SRBDs into consideration is universal, including scheduling, communications, patient flow, treatment, and continuing care.

BASIC PHYSIOLOGY

Appreciation of the impact SRBDs can have on dental practice is elevated when dental teams reflect that survival is based on 3 basic drives: hunger and thirst, sleep, and respiration. Of these, respiration is the most powerful; protecting the ability to breathe is the most important function of the autonomic nervous system. Anything that is done in the dental office that interferes with respiration is going to create bigger problems, anything that improves the body's ability to breathe may relieve challenges and allow physiologic systems to return to health. The state of health in the body is called homeostasis. Chronic disruption in basic health leads to long-term disease, termed somatic sensitization,[2] just like poor oral hygiene leads to increased dental disease. The more the dental team learns about the health impact of SRBD, the easier it will be to connect the current clinical evaluation with general health conditions and allow more important conversations between the dental office staff and the patient. A critical piece of data is how long the person has had SRBD because habits, physical adaptations, and physiologic effects have less impact the earlier in life they are redirected.

AIRWAY IMPACT ON NEW PATIENT ENCOUNTERS

The adult patient new to the dental practice is a clinical enigma with psychosocial, as well as physical, needs that must be addressed. They may not be prepared for questions about the airway at the dentist's office. Existing patients, handed new medical history forms or surveys about SRBD, may also be curious about this new line of inquiry from their trusted dental team. How the new questions are presented is critical. If the dental team does not explore the patient's thoughts and feelings about SRBD, the unanswered questions can hinder that trust, clouding the relationship and possibly interfering with accepting the doctor's recommended treatment plan. To keep the patients comfortable and gather accurate clinical information, every member of the dental team should be prepared to communicate why there are new screening questions. Systems must be created around the questions or else presentation, delivery, and discussion can severely disrupt patient flow. When the dental hygienist reports to the dentist that her patient has several risk factors for SRBD, it is up to the dentist to use that information while keeping the purpose of that preventive care visit in mind and inviting the patient for an additional visit to discuss these important findings.

The most important piece of information that the office can learn from the patient is the chief complaint, or the driving reason they are seeking medical services. Often, this is treated as a simple question and the cursory response is left unexplored. A much deeper relationship based on more important information can easily be started with a different system for learning why the patient contacted the office.

Do not ask a question such as "What brings you to our office today?" Ask, instead, "What in your life is worse because of the problems you are having?"

Do not ask, "What would you like to be different?" or "If you had a magic wand, what would you change?" Ask, instead, "How will your life improve when this problem is gone?"

If the patient has been prepared to think about the airway or is seeking specific SRBD therapy, encouraging him or her to talk about these questions will give the team much insight when it comes time for MDM and, later, for improving adherence to sometimes troublesome therapy. It allows a conversation beyond procedure or items (eg, cleaning or veneers) and connects overall health with the relationship-based dental team. There are 3 key elements:

- The team member who leads the conversation must be trained in verbal and relationship skills and recognize that the limiting factor is the patient's story, not the blanks on the form to be filled in or the time allocated for greeting a new patient.
- There must be a place in the office where a private conversations can be held.
- There must be a system for documenting key points so that others on the team can learn the details important to that patient as they move through treatment sequences.

TALK ABOUT THE PAST

People come to the dental office for dental services; therefore, even the most airway-focused general practice must address dental concerns. It is also human nature to begin to connect everything within one's world with a new, exciting, attention-grabbing subject. It is tempting to see SRBD problems with every dental concern. Although often justified, it requires discipline to focus on assessing the areas in which dental expertise is required. It is also true that, once becoming airway-aware, every clinical team member will see details never before noticed.

The next step in patient intake is the history of the present illness (HPI). The history enables the connections between SRBD and dental disease to start to become apparent because of screening questions such as the Epworth Sleepiness Scale and STOP-BANG (**Box 1**). If the patient has been diagnosed with bruxism, used a nightguard, had frequent headaches, or a history of cardiovascular disease, it is recorded in HPI. In medicine these are termed the problem list, review of systems, and impression. As part of the subjective, objective, assessment, and plan (SOAP) notes (**Box 2**), dental training labels these subjective.

Box 1
STOP-BANG screener for risk of obstructive sleep apnea

S: Do you snore loudly (louder than talking or loud enough to be heard through closed doors)?

T: Do you often feel tired, fatigued, or sleepy during the day?

O: Has anyone observed you not breathing during sleep?

P: Do you have or have you been treated for high blood pressure?

B: Is your body mass index more than 35 kg/m^2?

A: Is your age more than 50 years old?

N: Is your neck circumference greater than 15 inches (female patients) or 17 inches (male patients)?

G: Is your gender male?

You have a high risk of sleep apnea if you answered yes to 3 or more of the 8 STOP-BANG questions.

From Chung F, Abdullah HR, Liao P. STOP-Bang Questionnaire A Practical Approach to Screen for Obstructive Sleep Apnea. CHEST 2016; 149(3):631–8; with permission.

Box 2
SOAP

Subjective: what the patient says about their current condition

Objective: what the doctor finds during examination and results of tests

Assessment: the diagnosis

Plan: what the doctor recommends

It is during history that previous diagnoses and therapy attempts are detailed. The patient who has had a sleep test and tried other therapies (eg, positive airway pressure [PAP]) is quite different than the patient who shows signs of risk of an SRBD but has never been diagnosed. Part of it is simply asking and recording facts:

- What has improved the diagnosed disease?
- What makes it worse?
- How long has it been happening?
- What started it?
- What do they think should be done next?

By studying the format and details of these medical notes, the dental office's encounter notes can be improved. When requesting the notes from the patient's medical doctors, always ask for the full encounter notes because just getting the results of the sleep test leaves valuable information uncollected.

ASSESSMENT: THE PART DENTISTS ALREADY KNOW

Details of a thorough examination for oral health condition and recording of findings are not listed in this article. The dental team creates systems for gathering data for the licensed professional to use during MDM to create treatment recommendations for typical dental and periodontal therapy. Adding SRBD awareness disrupts these examination systems and requires the team to reformulate the data because MDM also must change. What have been thought of as oral health concerns might be caused by SRBDs.

AIRWAY IMPACT ON INFLAMMATORY DISEASES

Gingivitis and periodontal diseases arise from the body's reaction to pathogens, foreign bodies, or an injury to susceptible oral tissues, and become chronic when the inflammatory process does not return those tissues to homeostasis.[3] An SRBD, specifically obstructive sleep apnea, is accompanied by chronic intermittent hypoxemia and an increased circulating inflammatory response.[4] Adherence to dental preventive care is critical to control these diseases. If systemic challenges such as SRBD are left unaddressed, it can be frustrating to both the patient and clinician when management efforts fail. Patients with perpetually red gums or who struggle to resolve periodontal disease often protest, "I'm doing everything you tell me to do," and they may be right. The dental clinician who focuses only on flossing and brushing may find themselves disbelieving those patients, which is harmful to the professional relationship. Using more complicated, expensive, or troublesome methods of plaque control will more likely lead to a lack of adherence than successful management if the cause is left unaddressed. Patients who exhibit such unmanaged disease should be asked about airway-related issues. MDM about which therapy will promote homeostasis must involve reducing systemic inflammation. Dental hygienists who are airway-aware can be invaluable to help the patient connect the dots and seek more effective treatment.

If the dentist is thinking of using oral appliance therapy (OAT) for managing the airway, contraindications must be considered. As this information makes obvious, finding gingivitis or periodontitis is not a contraindication and, in fact, airway therapy may help. Of course, other considerations include deciding if the stability of the teeth is sufficient to anchor the device and if lip seal can be maintained to minimize drying of the tissue from mouth breathing. One reason that dentists are the only medical providers qualified to fit and manage OAT is their expertise in such therapeutic details.

MOUTH BREATHING

Mouth breathing and lack of lip coverage of the gingiva is known to increase inflammation in the gums[5] (**Fig. 1**). Other reasons why the tissue is not protected include insufficient nasal patency, enlarged adenoids and tonsils, and poor habits. The dental office is in the best position to lead therapy for chronic mouth breathing by addressing each of these areas.

Nasal patency can be enhanced with simple means, such as saline rinses, or use of inhaled glucocorticoids, such as fluticasone propionate.[6] Enlarged lymphoid tissues are addressed by otolaryngologists when referred by primary care physicians or dentists. Mouth breathing

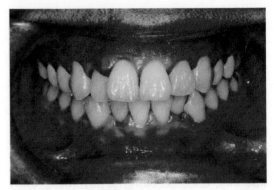

Fig. 1. Bright red gums from gingivitis due to mouth breathing are seen mostly on maxillary anterior teeth.

habits can be addressed in many ways.[7] One trend gaining popularity is encouraging lip seal during sleep with use of paper medical tape to hold the lips together. Patients often think they always breathe through their nose until mouth breathing is restricted, such as with OAT, and poor nasal patency may reduce adherence to appliance use. Links between mouth dryness and caries risk are well-established; improved nasal breathing, day and night, will enhance preventive efforts. Frequent office visits using agents such as artificial saliva, xylitol melts, or additional fluoride applications may be necessary for patients with extrinsic influences on saliva production, such as with many medications.

AIRWAY IMPACT ON THE TEETH

Enamel and dentin are not directly affected by airway problems; however, they can reflect disruptions to homeostasis resulting from SRBD. Teeth are afflicted by infection, acid attack, and forces that exceed their adaptive capacity.

CARIES

Tooth decay results from uncontrolled infection of the pellicle combined with susceptibility of the hard tooth structure to loss of mineralization.[8] The oral microbiome is complex and subject to influence by many factors, not just xerostomia.[9] What is important for the airway-aware dentist to keep in mind is the value of reducing mouth breathing, resulting in less challenge to the homeostasis of the oral environment. Placement of a custom device covering both arches of teeth will reduce salivary access to the teeth during the night. Because saliva production is normally reduced during sleep, counseling patients to place their clean and disinfected device over thoroughly cleaned teeth, perhaps with use of a fluoride rinse, before sleep, will minimize the impact of the acrylic device on caries incidence.

ACID EROSION

Acid can also come from sources outside the oral cavity. Discussion with patients about dietary choices, including acidic foods, is an important part of preventive care.[10] Gastroesophageal reflux (GER) is positively correlated with obesity and obstructive sleep apnea, although clinical cause and effect relationships are not completely understood.[11] Patients who are taking popular acid-reducing medications, such as the proton pump inhibitor omeprazole, may not think to discuss this with the dentist. Acid from GER causes a long list of symptoms and problems in the laryngopharynx and oral cavity, including tooth erosion.[12] Any finding of erosive lesions on the teeth should provoke a detailed discussion with the patient to identify the source of acid. Although occasional presence of acid in the mouth is easily felt, repeated dosing by acidic materials results in attenuated response.[13] Thus, the patient with chronic gastric acid in the mouth may not report any acidic sensation. It is entirely possible the dentist's examination and questioning may be the first time the patient has considered the possibility of GER disease (GERD) and referral to medical providers would be in order.

FORCE

When forces on teeth exceed the capacity of the periodontal support, mobility may result, which is classified as primary if the cause is periodontal disease or secondary if the support structures are healthy but the forces are more than they can bear. During the dental examination, the mobility of each tooth is assessed; however, the cautious dentist will wait to ascribe cause until all factors have been considered. As previously discussed, periodontal disease is partly a result of systemic inflammation, so a weakened bone support of teeth may result in mobility without an extra force such as bruxism. A search of the literature turns up hundreds of articles connecting mobility to factors far beyond the scope of this article. (See Alberto Herrero Babiloni and colleagues' article, "Transcranial Magnetic Stimulation: Potential Use in Obstructive Sleep Apnea and Sleep Bruxism," in this issue) Notably, a recent review of oral appliances for managing sleep bruxism found a greater decrease in bruxism with devices that protrude the mandible, improving sleep quality.[14] Occlusal

interferences and excessive tooth contact during parafunction produce wear facets on opposing teeth that are permanent unless reshaped or restored by a dentist. Facets might have formed years or decades before the examination, so their presence does not indicate current parafunctional activity.

ALIGNMENT OF THE OCCLUSION

The airway-aware dentist examines the shape of the dental arches to assess the skeletal base.

Thinking 3-dimensionally, the maxilla becomes the centerpiece for evaluating the interaction between teeth and airway. The width of the maxilla defines the shape of the palate and that, in turn, influences the nasal anatomy. When nasal airflow is restricted during the growth years (See Thomas Stark and colleagues' article, "Pediatric Considerations for Dental Sleep Medicine," in this issue), the maxilla is influenced to be narrow, with a high palatal vault, less room for the teeth, and a thicker and longer soft palate.[15] If the dentist were looking at such an arch form with only esthetics in mind, a narrow smile, empty buccal corridors, crowded teeth, or the need for extractions to satisfy orthodontic goals would be topics for discussion. If mandibular growth has been similarly restricted and is Angle class 2, significant occlusal instability may be present along with the esthetic issues. While talking about these concerns, the airway-focused dentist will link restricted arch forms to risk for SRBD and will take that into account during MDM. Patients expecting a plan for porcelain veneers might be surprised when the treatment options include correcting skeletal deficiencies. Adept use of communication skills will be necessary.[16]

Planning for occlusal therapy has traditionally focused on jaw joint function, occlusal muscle harmony, and force distribution across as many teeth as possible, detailing how teeth contact.[17] Because all of these can be influenced by an SRBD and therapy, the comprehensive approach takes airway into consideration at all levels of MDM. (See Thomas G. Schell's article, "Avoiding and Managing Oral Appliance Therapy Side Effects," and Noshir R. Mehta and Leopoldo P. Correa's article, "Oral Appliance Therapy and Temporomandibular Disorders," in this issue.)

AMERICAN DENTAL ASSOCIATION POLICY STATEMENT ON SLEEP-RELATED BREATHING DISORDERS

In 2018, the American Dental Association adopted a policy statement on the dentist's role in treating SRBD, establishing a set of expectations for the practice of dentistry.[18] Dentists are mandated to screen for SRBD in adults and children, and become familiar with local resources to direct at-risk patients for evaluation and therapy.

AIRWAY IMPACT ON DENTAL OFFICE SYSTEMS

Dental clinical encounters involve verbal and manual skills mastered by licensed professionals with the objective of prevention, management, and curing of disease. Provision of service requires many office systems to function efficiently. The dental team frequently changes these systems to accommodate a new material, instrument, team member, or schedule choice. Each change provokes a disruption in the system, which is necessary for improvement but often stressful to team members or even the business plan. When adding airway services, disruption can be far-reaching because new learning and new procedures accompany the need for examining nearly every office system.

The systems in any dental office are unique to the culture of the office: the dentists; the team; the physical facility; and, most of all, the leadership and communication of vision and goals. Understanding why the service mix is as it is determines the success of the practice.

Because systems vary widely, examining typical job positions in the dental office will illuminate functions, opportunities, and the effect airway therapy can have on the day-to-day operations. Creating smoothness in these operations can be reassuring to the people served, as well as the team. Patients can become uncomfortable with unfamiliar situations in which they will be asked to make important decisions based on the advice of the professionals they trust. Those patients with whom the most trust is established will feel confident in their decisions. A positive attitude about therapy choices always improves adherence and, ultimately, determines the success of the treatment.

FIRST CONTACT: THE TELEPHONE AND RECEPTION

People curious about airway therapy will call the office or ask the administrative staff for answers. Controlling this first impression is key to the ultimate success of the relationship. The person answering the phone must be keenly aware of the why airway therapy is necessary, the steps involved, and the best way to help the patient tell their story and their concerns. Existing patients are asked to return for an airway-focused discussion and new patients are invited to visit the office where they can experience the office culture. The best way to achieve this is to satisfy the patient's questions enough so they feel heard and valued but not so much that the caller feels no need to make an appointment. Listening carefully and responding with specific, thoughtful answers or additional questions will help the patient get to the point at which they request an appointment to meet the experts. Most people are not used to personalized encounters when calling a professional office. If they believe they are not being pressured to conform to office policy, the trust relationship will begin on a good note. Many of these skills are already well-known to the dental team; with the addition of airway-specific knowledge, applying relationship-building talents will fill the schedule with patients anxious to keep their appointments.

An example of a first contact might go something like this:

Caller: I can't use my CPAP [continuous PAP ventilator] and I heard you have a mouthpiece that can stop my snoring.

Scheduler: We're happy that our airway therapy has helped many people stop snoring, yes. Can you tell me more about your sleep breathing problem?

Caller: My wife made me go to the sleep clinic 2 years ago, they gave me a CPAP but I just can't use it. How much do the mouthpieces cost?

Scheduler: I'm sorry to hear that you still have a problem breathing well at night. Our doctor here is especially well trained to help people with your problem. The cost of therapy depends on several things. We're going to talk with you about that before you make any choices but it does depend on the doctor having a chance to do an examination first.

Caller: Can't you just tell me how much it will cost?

Scheduler: We'll be happy to discuss the cost of therapy when we've found out a little more about you. Is cost your biggest concern?

Caller: Not really, but I don't want to spend a lot of money if the mouthpiece isn't going to work.

Scheduler: There are more than 100 mouthpieces to choose from; our doctor can recommend which might give you the best night's sleep.

Caller: How does the doctor choose?

Scheduler: So that choice is best informed, our doctor will have to talk with you and complete a thorough examination here in the office.

Caller: When can I come in?

THE FIRST ENCOUNTER

No matter if your new airway patient is a long-standing dental patient or new to your office, the first time they visit to discuss SRBD, there will be new information needed during the check-in process. You will need to choose how you will interact with medical insurance. Although that is a big topic that requires more consideration than space allows here, you will be choosing whether you will participate with the patient in obtaining medical benefits or simply be providing your services for cash. Most patients will expect their medical problems to be covered by their medical insurance, so there is a requirement for the administrative team to be able to master either the process or the explanation for the cash-only choice. If you decide to help with insurance, the impact on your administrative systems is significant. Collecting benefit plan details, managing copayments, and looking online for medical benefit policies are all part of the work required. There are many professional billing service companies ready to help the dental office navigate these unfamiliar waters; however, engaging those services is, in itself, disruptive and will require significant effort and time commitment by the financial coordinator.

THE CLINICAL ENCOUNTER

Intake is the next step. The clinical team prepares the patient for the encounter with the doctor. During intake, vital signs are recorded, the HPI and review of systems are documented, and the patient is given the opportunity to ask questions about their diagnosis, history, and what the dentist can do. Nearly every bit of this sometimes time-consuming part of the encounter can be managed by well-trained team members. Systems will be needed to assemble records from other offices, such as encounter notes from physicians, sleep test results, and possibly radiographic images from other dentists. Typically, a clinical team member is designated and trained to complete the intake steps. Because personal health information is being discussed, intake is best done in a designated private space, such as a conference room. Scheduling and patient flow systems will need to be developed to allocate these physical and personnel resources.

The doctor then is invited to the encounter and the appropriate information summary is passed along by the clinical assistant. Asking about other concerns will help the patient feel heard and be able to tell the story important to them. With that background, the doctor can explore the chief complaint and provide answers to the patient's questions about treatment choices.

THE PHYSICAL EXAMINATION

Probably the least disrupted office system for airway therapy is the PE. Documentation now must include oropharyngeal and nasal airflow data. Recordings of oral health and disease will be specific about the impact of using a mandibular advancement device and which is the best choice.

ASSESSMENT AND PLAN

There is no system more affected by airway service than MDM, or treatment planning. The dentist, taking every part of the data into account, makes a recommendation for the next step to manage the airway problems diagnosed by the physician while keeping in mind the oral health management responsibilities available only in the dental office.

At this point, appropriate imaging is ordered. It must be determined whether a panoramic image will be sufficient or a cone-beam computed tomography (CBCT) image should be obtained. Each order (procedure, in dental-office jargon) must be backed by medical necessity. For every order, the clinical staff must document why it is needed. Often, patients with airway issues have histories of poor nasal airflow, chronic sinusitis, or temporomandibular disorder that bear investigating to support the provision of mandibular advancement therapy. The availability of CBCT technology allows a thorough assessment of the oral cavity and associated structures.

Dentists are the only experts in medicine who can make an assessment of teeth and supporting structures. The choice of whether a mandibular advancement device will be tolerable and safe for the patient, and which design is most suitable, is the responsibility of the trained dentist. This choice has yet to be successfully distilled into an algorithm to indicate the perfect device for a particular patient. MDM must take into account the previously discussed details and requires a bit of clinical wisdom to move forward. Because the context of the medical encounter always includes a patient with a diagnosis of obstructive sleep apnea, the medical risk is high. If due diligence is not undertaken, a poor match may result in low adherence or abandonment of therapy and ongoing risk of life-threatening disease. During MDM, it is always possible that the patient is not a good candidate for OAT and should be remanded to the physician for other treatment. Combination therapy and moving forward with OAT despite a poor prognosis are also well-established strategies, albeit ones that come with higher levels of oversight required because the airway management extends over months and years. Dentists used to a relatively rapid examination of dental disease, creation of a treatment plan, and getting on with treatment might find the impact of treating SRBD to be quite disruptive.

CHECKOUT AND FOLLOW-UP

Most dental treatment is fairly specific, with standard fees and follow-up, so production and collection percentages make sense. Fees are collected at time of service or by insurance payment according to schedules available to the financial administrative staff. Medical plans are not so predictable and there is always an element of uncertainty in medical benefits, despite the requirement of most for preauthorization and even office experience with other patients employed by the same workplace who are ostensibly covered by the same plan. Helping the patient accept this uncertainty falls to the financial staff and often they can benefit from enhanced verbal skills to smooth over what can be a difficult communications challenge. Having a private place in the office enhances the trust and security that facilitates these conversations.

Appointments required for SRBD therapy include

The initial examination
Records, after preauthorization, which device is chosen; images, scans, and impressions are obtained and sent to the laboratory.
Delivery
Follow-up at 1 week, 3 months, 6 months, and yearly, thereafter.[19]

Letters are sent to each of the patient's providers after the initial examination, delivery, and 3-month follow-up appointments, noting the patient's decisions, the therapy involved, and subjective results. Because these letters are customary, doctor and administrative systems must be created to produce and distribute them. Because all physicians use electronic records, they appreciate faxes, which can easily be incorporated into their charts, but most eschew email. No matter which format you choose, be sure the reports are short and to the point. Physicians care less about the details of each office visit than whether the patient is still in therapy and when they will be seeing the diagnosing physician next.

SUMMARY

Treating airway problems will increasingly fall to providers who do not have the extensive training of board-certified sleep physicians. Dentists are in a perfect position to have the most significant impact on community health by screening for and providing airway services appropriate to their training. This important work comes at a cost, however, to the normal function of a dental office focused on oral health. There are many new systems that must be developed that demand significant leadership skills to communicate value to the team. It is fortunate that the rewards that accompany the hard work of adapting to the new requirements are profound.

REFERENCES

1. Pankey LD, Davis WJ. A philosophy of the practice of dentistry. Toledo (OH): Medical College Press; 1985.
2. Gold AR. Functional somatic syndromes, anxiety disorders and the upper airway: a matter of paradigms. Sleep Med Rev 2010;15(6):389–401.
3. Hasturk H, Kantarci A. Activation and resolution of periodontal inflammation and its systemic impact. Periodontol 2000 2015;69:255–73.
4. Redline S, Yenokyan G, Gottlieb DJ, et al. Obstructive sleep apnea-hypopnea and incident stroke: the sleep heart health study. Am J Respir Crit Care Med 2010;182(2):269–77.
5. Wagaiyu EG, Ashley FP. Mouthbreathing, lip seal and upper lip coverage and their relationship with gingival inflammation in 11-14 year-old schoolchildren. J Clin Periodontol 1991;18(9): 698–702.
6. Bachert C, Pawankar R, Zhang L, et al. ICON chronic rhinosinusitis. World Allergy Organ J 2014; 7:25.
7. McKeown P. Close your mouth: Buteyko breathing clinic self-help manual. Galway (Ireland): Buteyko Books Loughwell; 2004.
8. Ismail AI, Pitts NB, Tellez M, et al. The International caries classification and management system (ICCMS™) an example of a caries management pathway. BMC Oral Health 2015;15(Suppl 1):S9.
9. Kaidonis J, Townsend G. The 'sialo-microbial-dental complex' in oral health and disease. Ann Anat 2016; 203:85–9.
10. Marshall TA. Dietary assessment and counseling for dental erosion. J Am Dent Assoc 2018;149(2): 148–52.
11. Akyüz F, Mutluay Soyer Ö. Which diseases are risk factors for developing gastroesophageal reflux disease? Turk J Gastroenterol 2017;28(Suppl 1): S44–7.
12. Gelardi M, Ciprandi G. Focus on gastroesophageal reflux (GER) and laryngopharyngeal reflux (LPR): new pragmatic insights in clinical practice.

J Biol Regul Homeost Agents 2018;32(1 Suppl. 2):41–7.

13. Wise PM, Wolf M, Thom SR, et al. The influence of bubbles on the perception carbonation bite. PLoS One 2013;8(8):e71488.

14. Jokubauskas L, Baltrušaitytė A, Pileičikienė G. Oral appliances for managing sleep bruxism in adults: a systematic review from 2007 to 2017. J Oral Rehabil 2018;45(1):81–95.

15. Gungor AY, Turkkahraman H. Effects of airway problems on maxillary growth: a review. Eur J Dent 2009; 3(3):250–4.

16. Young LB, O'Toole C, Wolf B. Communication skills for dental health care providers. Park (IL): Quintessence; 2015.

17. Dawson PE. Evaluation, diagnosis, and treatment of occlusal problems. 2nd edition. St Louis (MO): Mosby; 1989.

18. Policy statement on the role of dentistry in the treatment of sleep-related breathing disorders. American Dental Association; 2018. Available at: www.ada.org.

19. American Academy of Dental Sleep Medicine AADSM treatment protocol: oral appliance therapy for sleep disordered breathing: an update for 2013.

Pediatric Considerations for Dental Sleep Medicine

Thomas R. Stark, LTC, DDS[a],*, Manuel Pozo-Alonso, COL, DDS[b], Raj Daniels, MAJ, MD[c], Macario Camacho, MAJ, MD[d]

KEYWORDS

- Obstructive sleep apnea • Pediatric OSA • Dental sleep medicine • OSA management
- Rapid maxillary expansion

KEY POINTS

- Pediatric OSA differs from adult OSA in both diagnosis and management. OSA in children is a common health problem with unique cardiovascular, metabolic, and neurocognitive consequences.
- Dentists are well-positioned to recognize pediatric risk factors for OSA. Signs and symptoms of OSA may be noticed by dental professionals during the patient interview, clinical examination, and while performing dental treatment.
- Medical treatment is not always successful or indicated for pediatric patients with OSA. Dentists may provide valuable alternative and adjunctive treatment options for pediatric OSA.
- Rapid maxillary expansion (RME) is indicated for treating some cases of OSA. RME involves orthopedic expansion of the midpalatal suture to correct posterior crossbites, improve facial symmetry, decrease nasal resistance, and increase airway volume.
- Pediatric OSA is a complicated medical condition. Interdisciplinary treatment involving medical and dental professionals may optimize care and improve the durability of OSA treatment.

Disclaimer: The opinions or assertions contained herein are the private ones of the authors and are not to be construed as official or reflecting the view of the US Army, the Uniformed Services University of the Health Sciences or the Department of Defense. None of the authors have a financial interest in any commercial product or service discussed in this work.

Disclosures: None.

Funding: No funding was received for this research.

Conflict of Interest: All authors certify that they have no affiliations with or involvement in any organization or entity with any financial interest (such as honoraria; educational grants; participation in speakers' bureaus; membership, employment, consultancies, stock ownership, or other equity interest; and expert testimony or patent-licensing arrangements), or nonfinancial interest (such as personal or professional relationships, affiliations, knowledge, or beliefs) in the subject matter or materials discussed in this article.

Consent for this Study: Consent forms were obtained for clinical photos. There is no identifying information included in this article.

Ethical Approval: This article has not been presented at a meeting. All procedures performed in studies involving human participants were in accordance with the ethical standards of the institutional and/or national research committee and with the 1964 Helsinki declaration and its later amendments or comparable ethical standards.

[a] Uniformed Service Health Science University, Departments of Pediatric Dentistry and Orofacial Pain, Dental Health Activity Rheinland Pfalz, APO, AE 09005, Wiesbaden, Germany; [b] Uniformed Service Health Science University, Department of Orthodontics, Dental Health Activity Rheinland Pfalz, Landstuhl 09180, Germany; [c] Uniformed Service Health Science University, Department of Pediatrics, Division of Sleep Medicine, Tripler Army Medical Center, 1 Jarrett White Road, Honolulu 96859, Hawaii; [d] Uniformed Service Health Science University, Division of Otolaryngology, Head and Neck Surgery, Tripler Army Medical Center, 1 Jarrett White Road, Honolulu 96859, Hawaii

* Corresponding author.

E-mail address: trstark@gmail.com

Sleep Med Clin 13 (2018) 531–548
https://doi.org/10.1016/j.jsmc.2018.08.002
1556-407X/18/© 2018 Elsevier Inc. All rights reserved.

INTRODUCTION

Obstructive sleep apnea (OSA) is defined as a disorder of breathing during sleep characterized by prolonged partial upper airway obstruction and/or intermittent complete obstruction that disrupts normal ventilation during sleep and normal sleep patterns.[1] Pediatric OSA differs from adult OSA and in some cases can be a serious medical condition with unique characteristics, diagnosis, and management, recommendations.[2] Dentists have a well-established position in the management of OSA in adult patients.[3] However, the place of dentists in management of pediatric OSA is not as clear.[4] Dental sleep medicine is an emerging field and the role of dental professionals in the management of pediatric patients is gaining considerable attention.[5] This paper aims to discuss the important role dentists have in identifying and assisting with the management of OSA in children.

SLEEP-RELATED BREATHING DISORDERS

Sleep-related breathing disorders (SRBDs) are on a continuum ranging from the benign and intermittent snoring to the more morbid severe sleep apnea (**Table 1**).[6] Sleep apneas are categorized as obstructive, central, or mixed respiratory events. Obstructive apneas occur due to a partial or complete obstruction in the upper airway while central apneas occur because the central nervous system fails to trigger ventilation.

OBSTRUCTIVE SLEEP APNEA DEFINED

OSA involves partial or complete blockage of airflow while sleeping.[6] For pediatric patients, apnea refers to complete cessation of airflow (by at least 90% compared with baseline) for at least the duration of 2 breaths during baseline breathing 10 seconds. Hypopnea in pediatric patients refers to airflow reduction (by at least 30% compared with baseline) for at least the duration of 2 breaths during baseline breathing accompanied by either at least 3% oxygen desaturation or an arousal from sleep.[6] The apnea hypopnea index (AHI) refers to the number of apneas plus the number of hypopneas observed per hour during a sleep study.[6]

OBSTRUCTIVE SLEEP APNEA CONSIDERATIONS

The upper airway is a pliable tube spanning from the nasal cavity and hard palate to the vocal cords that increases in collapsibility during sleep.[7] Collapse of the upper airway can result in oxygen desaturation. Because oxygen is essential for life, pediatric OSA has been associated with

Table 1
Sleep related breathing disorder categories*

Categories	Conditions	Pediatric Significance
Isolated symptoms and normal variants	Snoring Catathrenia	• May be initial indication of sleep-related breathing disorder
Obstructive sleep apnea (OSA) disorders	OSA	• Pediatric OSA defined as younger than 18 years old • American Academy of Sleep Medicine (AASM) manual states adult criteria may be used for patients older than 13 years • Snorting, gasping, and choking at night is OSA until proven otherwise • Continuous positive airway pressure (CPAP) use has rarely been associated with malocclusion and midface hypoplasia • May be candidates for dental interventions • Increased sedation risks
Central sleep apnea (CSA) syndromes	Primary CSA (includes CSA in infancy and prematurity) Secondary CSA (high altitude, medical condition, substance or medication, treatment emergent)	• CPAP use has rarely been associated with malocclusion and midface hypoplasia • Not candidates for dental interventions • Increased sedation risks

* Sleep-related hypoventilation and sleep-related hypoxemia not included.

pulmonary, cardiovascular, inflammatory, metabolic, and neurocognitive consequences.[8]

Cardiovascular Complications

Circulating inflammatory mediators, endothelial dysfunction, and intermittent abnormalities in gas exchange are likely responsible for many of the negative consequences of pediatric OSA.[9] Because children have less functional oxygen reserve than adults, they can quickly develop hypercapnia and hypoxia. Consequently, even short episodes of apnea can result in severe hypoxemia.[8] Lack of oxygen during sleep induces a physiologic phenomenon known as hypoxic pulmonary vasoconstriction.[10] Low oxygen or hypoxia causes small arteries in the lungs to constrict. This in turn raises the pressure of the lung's arteries and can lead to a condition known as pulmonary hypertension.[10] As a result, abnormal enlargement of the right side of the heart or cor pulmonale may occur.[11] Pediatric OSA also has been associated with elevated systemic blood pressure and sinus arrythmias.[6,12]

Metabolic Complications

Pediatric OSA has been associated with metabolic and endocrine disorders.[13] Growing children have higher metabolic rates than adults. Growth hormone secretion peaks during deep sleep (slow wave sleep: stage 3).[13] For this reason, increases in height and weight have been observed following adenotonsillectomy in children with OSA.[14,15] Interestingly, this has been demonstrated in both a normal population and in children with failure to thrive.[14,16] Hormonal pathways and energy expenditure at night are likely related to growth considerations in children.[16,17] Data suggest that pediatric OSA is related to insulin sensitivity and metabolic syndrome.[14] However, some studies find that insulin resistance is more likely related to obesity than OSA.[18]

Behavioral and Neurocognitive Complications

Fragmentation of sleep and episodic hypoxia are likely related to behavioral health neurocognitive consequences.[19] Behavioral manifestations of OSA in pediatric patients may differ from adults. Similar to adults, some children may complain of sleepiness, whereas others may demonstrate hyperactivity, inattentiveness, aggressiveness, or even symptoms of depression.[20] Sleep fragmentation influences the ventrolateral prefrontal cortex, the area of the brain responsible for the control of affect and prolonged concentration and attention.[20] As such, OSA has been associated with academic underperformance in schoolchildren.[21,22]

Autonomic arousal, activation of the reticular formation of the brain, and increased body movements may occur in children with OSA.[20] Data from polysomnography (PSG) demonstrates that children with OSA have fewer cortical activations than adults.[6] Moreover, children also tend to have fewer disruptions in sleep architecture.[6]

EPIDEMIOLOGY OF SLEEP-RELATED BREATHING DISORDERS

Intermittent snoring occurs in up to 20% of children, whereas regular snoring has been reported to occur in at a rate 7% to 10%.[22,23] Studies suggest a 1% to 4% prevalence of OSA in pediatric patients.[24] Despite increased awareness in the adult population, OSA often goes unrecognized in infants, children, and teens.[24] Infants born premature are more likely to have OSA.[20] OSA occurs equally in young boys and girls; however, data suggest adolescent OSA is more common in boys than girls.[25,26]

Tonsils and adenoids enlarge progressively from age 2 to 8 years and are largest in relation to airway between ages 3 and 6 years making this an important period for OSA.[27] Lymphoid tissues decrease in size in adolescence.[27] However, the potential for obesity and possible role of sex hormones may explain this secondary peak period of OSA for teens and emerging adults.[28]

RISK FACTORS FOR PEDIATRIC OBSTRUCTIVE SLEEP APNEA

A number conditions and factors predispose pediatric patients to the development of OSA. Identification of risk factors for SRBD may alert clinicians to make timely referrals.

Physical Airway Obstruction

Adenotonsillar hypertrophy is the main cause of OSA in children; however, the potential for airway obstruction occurs at several levels.[29] Blockages of the nasopharyngeal airway, such as choanal atresia or turbinate hypertrophy, contribute by reducing airflow through the pharyngeal passages. Macroglossia impacts airway dynamics by encroaching on retroglossal and retropalatal space.[29] The epiglottis and supraglottis represent additional regions of potential obstruction.[30,31] Hypotonia, as is seen in muscular dystrophies and cerebral palsy, leads to increased generalized collapsibility of the airway.[32]

Craniofacial Anomalies and Malocclusions

Craniofacial anomalies and skeletal malocclusions, such as mandibular or maxillomandibular deficiency, are consistently related to OSA.[33] A systematic review of craniofacial morphologic and orthodontic characteristics in pediatric patients with OSA include high palatal vault, narrow maxillary arch, posterior crossbite, long lower anterior face height, steep gonial angle, posterior-inferior rotation of the mandible, vertical and clockwise growth pattern, retrusive chin, lip incompetence, and smaller nasopharyngeal airway spaces.[33]

Obesity

As with adults, obesity is a risk factor for pediatric OSA.[18] However, most young children with OSA are not obese.[27] Nonetheless, a recent study found that obesity was a better indicator of OSA than snoring in middle school children.[34]

Premature Birth

Premature birth is another important risk factor for OSA.[20] It has been hypothesized that differences in feeding, swallowing, and anatomic findings, such as high arching narrow palate, are reasons for the connection between prematurity and SRBD.[35]

Other Factors

Several other factors may be related to OSA. Exposure to second-hand smoke is an example of an environmental risk factor. In contrast, adolescents who smoke do not appear to be at an increased risk for OSA.[33] African American ethnicity, Hispanic ethnicity, residency in disadvantaged neighborhoods, and history of upper and lower respiratory disease have been associated with OSA in children.[25,36,37]

SIGNS AND SYMPTOMS OF OBSTRUCTIVE SLEEP APNEA

As with adults, children with OSA may present with symptoms of daytime sleepiness, difficulty waking in the mornings, and morning headaches. Pediatric patients may present with hyperactivity, difficulty with school, depressed mood, and inattentiveness.[6] Given these points, patients may be mistakenly categorized as lazy or defiant. In fact, pediatric OSA may be mistakenly diagnosed with behavioral health conditions, such as attention deficit disorder or attention deficit hyperactivity disorder.[38]

Several visible and audible features present with pediatric OSA. Snoring, snorting, gasping, and choking sounds may be heard during sleep. Sleep bruxism also may be present.[6] Hyponasal speech may be an awake audible clue.[28] It is important to recognize that hyponasal differs from hypernasal speech. In hyponasal speech, the patient sounds congested because the patient cannot breathe well through the nose. On the contrary, hypernasal is related to increased nasal airflow, which is more common in patients with velopharyngeal insufficiency, such as a patient with cleft palate.

Observable features during sleep include observed apneic pause, sweating during sleep, paradoxic chest wall movement, fitful sleep, sleep bruxism, and sleeping with neck hyperextended or other unusual position.[6] Parents also may describe confused arousals.[19] Mouth breathing, allergic shiners, and Dennie-Morgan folds are common in patients with allergic rhinitis and may also present with OSA.[39] Last, there is an association with OSA and nocturnal enuresis (NE).[40]

Sleep Bruxism and Obstructive Sleep Apnea

Sleep bruxism is a sleep-related movement disorder that has been associated with SRBDs in children.[41] Sleep bruxism is defined as "repetitive jaw muscle activity characterized by clenching or grinding of the teeth and/or bracing or thrusting of the mandible."[6] Diagnostic criteria for sleep bruxism include regular or frequent tooth grinding sounds occurring during sleep along with the presence of either abnormal tooth wear or transient morning jaw muscle pain or fatigue, and/or jaw locking on awakening.[6] Sleep bruxism peaks during childhood and decreases with age. The prevalence of sleep bruxism is frequently reported in 14% to 17% in children.[6] The pathophysiology of sleep bruxism is not well understood and the etiology is unclear. Although sleep bruxism is common and may not be related to any other condition, it also has been associated with attention deficit hyperactivity disorder, gastroesophageal reflux, and several other psychological and medical conditions.[6]

DIAGNOSIS OF OBSTRUCTIVE SLEEP APNEA

According to the 2014 third edition of the International Classification for Sleep Disorders, diagnosis of pediatric OSA is based on a combination of subjective characteristics along with sleep laboratory findings (**Box 1**).[6] Polysomnography is required for the diagnosis of OSA in both children and adults. Sleep laboratories should have proficiency in managing pediatric patients, as diagnosis of pediatric OSA differs from adult OSA. Sleep studies are somewhat invasive and intimidating and require patient cooperation.

Although pediatric OSA was defined in 1976, there has been much debate regarding

---

Box 1
Obstructive sleep apnea, pediatric

Diagnostic Criteria

Criteria A and B must be met

A. The presence of one or more of the following:

   1. Snoring.

   2. Labored, paradoxical, or obstructed breathing during the child's sleep.

   3. Sleepiness, hyperactivity, behavioral problems, or learning problems.

B. PSG demonstrates one or both of the following:

   1. One or more obstructive apneas, mixed apneas, or hypopneas, per hour of sleep.

      OR

   2. A pattern of obstructive hypoventilation, defined as at least 25% of total sleep time with hypercapnia ($PaCO_2$ > 50 mm Hg) in association with one or more of the following:

      a. Snoring.

      b. Flattening of the inspiratory nasal pressure waveform.

      c. Paradoxical thoracoabdominal motion.

Notes

1. Respiratory events defined according to the most recent version of the AASM Manual for the Scoring of Sleep and Associated Events.

---

diagnosis and scoring criteria in children.[42] The threshold for apneas and hypoxias in children is less than for adults. The AHI may vary between studies based on the scoring criteria used. The American Association of Sleep Medicine established scoring criteria in 2007. Across studies, apneas tend to be measured consistently; however, there is significant variability with hypopneas. There is a lack of well-defined criteria to identify respiratory effort–related arousals; therefore, there is considerable variability in PSG interpretation.[41] Subsequently, patients may be underdiagnosed or overdiagnosed with pediatric OSA. A recent study indicates that current scoring criteria underscore pediatric SRBD.[42] Some institutions use 3% desaturation scoring criteria, which provides increased sensitivity in detecting OSA, whereas other institutions use Medicare guidelines, which use 4% desaturation scoring criteria with increased specificity.

CENTRAL SLEEP APNEA

Central sleep apnea (CSA) differs from OSA in that there is a lack of respiratory effort during periods of oxygen desaturation. Ventilation is controlled by centers in the brainstem and carbon dioxide is required to trigger ventilation. Skeletal anomalies leading to brainstem compression and chronic kidney disease secondary and alterations in respiratory control due to chronic kidney disease are examples of medical conditions related to CSA.[43] Medications, such as opioids and benzodiazepines, are associated with CSA, because they interfere with respiratory drive.

PEDIATRIC DENTAL SLEEP MEDICINE

Dentists are in a favorable position to recognize, make appropriate medical referrals, and support the medical team in the management of sleep-related breathing conditions. Although awareness of OSA and sleep-disordered breathing is high among pediatric dentists, a recent study demonstrated that screening is not standard or commonly provided.[44] There are 3 main ways dentists can gather information related to SRBDs: (1) patient interview and screening, (2) clinical examination, and (3) observances during dental treatment.

Patient Interview and Screening

The initial examination provides an ideal opportunity for uncovering risk factors associated with pediatric OSA. Direct questioning about history of PSG or treatment for sleep disorders is one method of obtaining information. Asking the parent to complete a health history form in which they may select sleep-disordered breathing, such as snoring or OSA, from a list of medical conditions is another approach. History of premature birth also places a child at an increased risk for having OSA. Medical diagnoses commonly associated with OSA include Trisomy 21, muscular dystrophy, collagen disorders, sickle cell disease, and several other craniofacial disorders and syndromes (**Table 2**).

A screening instrument known as BEARS (B = Bedtime, E = Excessive Daytime Sleepiness, A = Night Awakenings, R = Regularity and duration of sleep, S = Snoring) has been used in primary care settings to gain more information about sleep.[45] Alternatively, asking screening questions about snoring, witnessed apneas, mouth breathing at night, enuresis, hyperactivity, difficulty concentrating, academic performance, and sleep bruxism provides useful information about sleep. Children may provide accurate

Table 2
Medical conditions associated with pediatric obstructive sleep apnea (OSA)

Conditions Associated with OSA	Likely Mechanism
Down syndrome	Enlarged tongue, hypotonia, short neck, midface hypoplasia, tendency toward obesity
Neuromuscular disease • Muscular dystrophies • Myotonias • Neuropathies	Hypotonia
Cerebral palsy	Hypotonia
Marfan	Excessive tissue laxity leading to collapsible airway
Mucopolysaccharide storage diseases • Hurler syndrome • Scheie syndrome • Sly syndrome	Accumulation of macromolecules in upper airway tissue
Achondroplasia	Midface hypoplasia, short cranial base
Craniosynostosis • Apert • Crouzon • Pfeiffer	Midface hypoplasia May have comorbid central sleep apnea due to brainstem compression
Pierre Robin sequence	Cleft, high arched palate, micrognathia, retrognathia, glossoptosis
Craniofacial microsomia • Goldenhar • Hemifacial macrosomia • First and second brachial arch syndrome	Retruded mandible
Mandibulofacial dysostosis • Treacher Collins	Mandibular deficiency Cleft palate
Other craniofacial syndromes • CHARGE • Stickler • Hallermann-Streiff	Combination of skeletal factors
Beckwith-Weideman	Macroglossia, obesity
Prader-Willi	Obesity, hypotonia
Sickle cell disease	Reduced upper airway patency and adenotonsillar hypertrophy
Postpharygoplasty	Airway changes
Klippel-Feil	C-spine abnormalities may cause airway narrowing
Cleft lip and palate	Smaller airway Disrupted oropharyngeal musculature

answers if they are old enough; however, most validated sleep screeners are based on parent response.[46]

Clinical Examination

A thorough clinical examination may prompt medical referrals if a pediatric SRBD is suspected. Coupled with information from the patient interview, patients with venous pooling beneath the eyes or a characteristic long adenoid facies may warrant further evaluation.[39] However, these are nonspecific findings and may be present in healthy controls and patients with other conditions, such as seasonal allergies.[39] The Mallampati and tonsil hypertrophy scores provide further information about the oropharyngeal airway (**Fig. 1**). Dry lips and erythematous and edematous maxillary gingiva are possibly related to nighttime mouth breathing.[35] Maxillary constriction, narrow or V-shaped palate, low tongue posture, ankyloglossia, and retroglossal airway narrowing have been associated with OSA in the pediatric population.[4] Retrognathic profile, excessive overjet, and posterior crossbite may indicate airway issues.[4,33]

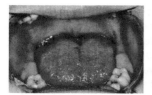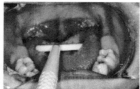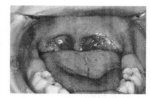

Fig. 1. If the airway is not easily observable, a mirror or tongue blade may be used to assist with visualization. Note the airway obstruction caused by the tonsils and uvula in this young child.

Observances During Dental Treatment

Dental treatment is another opportunity for dental practitioners to recognize potential sleep-related breathing problems. The airway is often well visualized while the patient is in a semi-reclined position during dental treatment. The dentist can observe a patient's ability to breath freely through the nose during dental procedures. Snoring may be directly observed if a patient doses off during dental treatment. If nitrous oxide or sedation is used, partial or complete airway obstructions may become even more obvious. Use of a pretracheal or precordial stethoscope is helpful for identifying air movement and alerting the practitioner to airway obstruction. Patients with OSA have an increased risk for adverse outcomes during sedation.[45,47] Opioid analgesics used as sedative medications can cause central apneas to occur as well. Rescue airway equipment should be available to bypass obstructions and providers should be prepared to assist with oxygenation and ventilation if necessary.

OBSTRUCTIVE SLEEP APNEA TREATMENT CONSIDERATIONS
Defining Treatment Success

There are also limitations when it comes to defining successful treatment of OSA in children. Subjective improvement in symptoms may not be reliable and night-to-night variability of PSGs is another concern. OSA is multifactorial, and changes in weight or growth and development may also impact treatment course.

Subjective measures of success include improvements in OSA symptoms, such as sleepiness and behavior. Improved performance in school is another factor that may be used to determine treatment success. Subjective improvement may not correlate with resolution of OSA.

Success is often categorized objectively as improvement in PSG parameters; however, these variables also may fluctuate. AHI and SPO_2 nadir or lowest oxygen saturation (LSAT) are often used as to measure treatment outcome in OSA. An AHI of zero is ideal; however, less than 1 is considered within normal limits for children. Improvements in LSAT or oxygen desaturation index (ODI) are commonly used as a measure of successful treatment in pediatric OSA.

TREATMENT OPTIONS
Soft Tissue Surgery

Adenotonsillectomy is the most common recommendation for children with OSA. Other soft tissue surgeries may be appropriate if the nasopharyngeal or oropharyngeal airway is compromised.[48,49] The Childhood Adenotonsillectomy Trial (CHAT) was introduced to determine the advantages of adenotonsillectomy over watchful waiting for children with uncomplicated OSA.[50] This randomized controlled study demonstrated improvements in sleep apnea symptoms, daytime behavior, subjective sleepiness, and quality of life.[51] However, the trial did not support any changes in executive cognitive function after surgery.[52] Relapse of OSA is not uncommon after adenotonsillectomy.[53] Indeed, a systematic review and meta-analysis found that only 59.8% of children were cured of OSA (based on AHI of <1) following tonsillectomy and adenoidectomy.[53] Residual OSA is more common in teenagers and in cases of severe OSA before surgery.[54] Children with obesity, asthma, craniofacial abnormalities, and neurologic/developmental abnormalities also have a high risk of residual OSA.[54]

Orthognathic Surgery

Orthognathic surgery is another option in cases of severe skeletal malocclusion or medically refractory OSA.[55] Distraction osteogenesis using internal or external rigid fixation is another surgical approach for pediatric patients with retrognathia.[31,56] Maxillomandibular advancement is the gold standard for orthognathic surgery.[57] Due to growth concerns, some surgeons prefer to wait until late teen years for girls and early 20s for boys.[57] Mandibular advancement and surgically assisted rapid palatal expansion are additional orthognathic surgery options. Jackson[58] reported a case of a 16-year-old with residual OSA who received bilateral sagittal split osteotomy and mandibular advancement. Subjective symptoms along with improvements in AHI, ODI, and sleep architecture were noted. Orthognathic surgery has potential for relapse and other complications.[59]

Positive Airway Pressure Therapy

Positive airway pressure therapy is indicated when surgery is contraindicated or while a patient is awaiting surgical intervention. Continuous positive airway pressure (CPAP) or bilevel positive airway pressure is often used in cases in which OSA persists following surgery.[60] Studies suggest CPAP compliance is variable, ranging from 49% to 70%.[61,62] Parental reports often overestimate CPAP adherence.[61] Female sex and developmental delay were associated with better adherence.[62] Of note, nasal CPAP may have orthodontic implications because it may alter midface growth.[63]

Medications

A trial of intranasal corticosteroids may be appropriate for some cases of pediatric OSA.[64,65] Intranasal steroids can potentially reduce the size of hypertrophic adenotonsilar tissues, thereby improving nasal airflow. Intranasal fluticasone and budesonide may reduce OSA severity.[64,65] Intranasal corticosteroids require compliance and adherence to daily use because the effects are not immediate. Montelukast is a systemic leukotriene modifier that reduces OSA severity in children.[66,67]

Oropharyngeal Exercises (Myofunctional Therapy)

Oral exercises have been reported to have a positive impact on SRBD.[35] Myofunctional therapy is described by Moeller and colleagues[68] as "treatment of dysfunctions of the muscles of the face and mouth, with the purpose of correcting orofacial functions, such as chewing and swallowing, and promoting nasal breathing." Although the mechanism of action is not well understood, oral exercises may increase tone of the genioglossus muscle.[68] It is hypothesized that increased tone may relate to fewer episodes of airway obstruction during sleep. Oropharyngeal exercises have been associated with a reduction in OSA symptoms, increased oxygen saturation, and increased oral breathing.[69]

Oral breathing influences palatal development in growing children.[70] Underdeveloped midface, transverse maxillary deficiency, and palatal constriction are commonly associated with children who are oral breathers.[71] Guilleminault and Huang[72] report that myofunctional reeducation may be introduced early in life to engage primitive reflexes present at birth, discourage mouth breathing, and use continuous nose breathing whether awake or asleep. In addition to use in growing patients, data also suggest that myofunctional therapy may serve as a useful adjunctive treatment to improve durability of surgical therapy for OSA.[73]

ORTHODONTIC AND DENTOFACIAL ORTHOPEDIC TREATMENT

Oral appliances have been recognized by the medical community as a useful treatment option for the management of OSA in adults.[3] Oral appliances or mandibular advancement devices (MADs) hold the mandible in an anterior position during sleep.

By the same token, orthodontic appliances also have important considerations. Orthodontic treatment not only creates favorable occlusal and skeletal relationships, but also impacts airway dynamics.

Functional Appliances

Orthodontists have used functional appliances in growing children as an early dentofacial orthopedic intervention. A systematic review and meta-analysis on the use of functional appliances in growing children with class II malocclusions demonstrated radiographic evidence of increased oropharyngeal dimensions when compared with controls.[74] Increased airway space may decrease nasal resistance and have a positive impact on OSA.[75]

In select cases, functional repositioning of the mandible may lead to an improvement in childhood OSA.[76] Functional appliances aimed at "growing" mandibles have been a subject of much controversy and debate. Although early mandibular growth has been demonstrated with functional appliance use, data suggest the final size of the mandible is approximately the same size as it would have been without any treatment.[77,78]

Mandibular Advancement Devices

MADs are removable functional appliances worn while sleeping. A 2016 Cochrane review found insufficient evidence to support or refute the use of oral appliances to manage OSA in children.[76] Case reports and small sample studies demonstrate efficacy in select cases.[76] A randomized crossover clinical trial found clinically relevant reduction in supine AHI in children.[79] Evidence for MAD in children is limited, and long-term outcomes on safety and efficacy are unavailable.[80] However, short-term resolution of OSA may be observed with the use of MAD in children and adolescents.[80]

PALATAL CONSTRICTION

Narrow palatal anatomy may occur with or without a posterior crossbite. Crossbites may be dental, skeletal, or a combination. Simple dental crossbites involve the teeth only, whereas skeletal crossbites are associated with a narrow palate and compensatory mandibular shift.[81]

Posterior Crossbite with Functional Shift

Unilateral posterior crossbites with habitual shifts are associated with growth asymmetries.[82] Ultrasound studies have confirmed the presence of asymmetry of masseter muscles in growing children with posterior crossbites and functional shifts.[83] In a like manner, condylar asymmetry also may occur.[84] For these reasons, posterior crossbites with functional mandibular shifts should be corrected as early as feasibly possible.[81] A considerable benefit of early expansion includes potential avoidance of surgical expansion in the future. However, orthognathic surgery is ideal for some patients.

PALATAL EXPANSION
Rapid Maxillary Expansion or Rapid Palatal Expansion

Orthopedic expansion of the maxilla widens the hard palate, raises the soft palate, broadens the nasal passages, and can be considered for the management of OSA.[82] McNamara and colleagues[82] describe rapid maxillary expansion (RME) as an "effective orthopedic procedure used to treat structural and functional problems in the midface." RME involves application of lateral orthopedic forces at the immature midpalatal suture. During this incremental process, bone fills in the gap between the displaced segments.[84] Once ideal expansion is achieved, retention is accomplished by leaving an orthodontic appliance in place for a period of time as the new bone matures and consolidates.[85] This process of gradually lengthening bones is known as distraction osteogenesis and has been used by orthopedic specialists for more than a century.

Cistulli and colleagues[86] first introduced RME as a treatment option for OSA in a 1998 pilot study. A reduction in AHI was noted in the patients treated with RME. Subsequent studies support expansion as an effective treatment option for some cases of OSA.[87–89] A recent systematic review and meta-analysis revealed an overall reduction in AHI following RME therapy in children.[90] Another systematic review and meta-analysis on rapid palatal expansion for pediatric OSA demonstrated an improvement in lowest oxygen saturation, and AHI was consistently noted in the short term (less than 3 years).[91] Pooled data from 313 patients demonstrated a mean LSAT increase from 87.0% ± 9.1% to 96.0% ± 2.7% and a 70.0% reduction in AHI.[91] Long-term resolution stability and maintenance have been demonstrated after expansion.[92]

Currently there are no randomized controlled studies demonstrating the treatment effect of RME on OSA. Therefore, it is possible that some of the cases of OSA resolved spontaneously or were due to normal growth changes.[93]

The following are 3 potential ways RME assists patients with OSA: (1) nasal airway changes, (2) oropharyngeal airway changes, and (3) mandibular positioning and growth changes.

Nasal airway changes

RME may be associated with increases nasal space, reduction in nasal resistance, and improvement in respiratory patterns.[94,95] A 2015 consensus paper by McNamara and colleagues[82] concluded that an orthopedic expansion of the maxilla provides a stable and significant increase in upper airway volume in the maxillary and nasopharyngeal regions. Cone-beam computed tomography (CBCT) is an important tool for analyzing airway volume expansion.[96,97] A systematic review of CBCT studies and RME therapy reported inconsistencies in CBCT protocols for nasal volume measurement.[98] Although commonly used in research, the assessment of airway changes using 3-dimensional radiographic imaging techniques should not be routinely performed in children.[99]

Data consistently demonstrate improvements in nasal resistance following RME. Reduction of nasal obstruction appears to be an important factor in the improvement in OSA in children.[97] Nasal airway obstructions may be evaluated using fiberoptic endoscopy.[100] Nasal airway resistance is measured and overall nasal airflow is measured using standard rhinomanometry or acoustic rhinometry.[100] These diagnostic tools are used to measure and assess airway resistance before and after RME therapy.[94,99] Computer modeling and computational fluid dynamics simulations are used in research settings to provide a more detailed assessment of nasal airway ventilation.[95,101]

Oropharyngeal airway changes

Maxillary expansion transforms a high, narrow, "v"-shaped palate to more shallow, broad and "u"-shaped counterpart. Although RME intuitively provides more room in the mouth for the tongue, data suggest the oropharyngeal dimensions may actually remain unchanged. To that point, studies suggest that oropharyngeal volume may not increase following RME even when OSA is effectively treated.[97,102,103] However, a study by Fastuca and colleagues[104] demonstrated increase in total airway volume following RME. It is important to realize the tongue represents the anterior portion of the collapsible airway. Changes in the oropharyngeal spaces are complicated and may be related to several factors, such as tongue position.

Indirect changes in static tongue posture represent a potential advantage of RME. Expansion appears to be associated with a raised tongue posture, which may be advantageous with OSA. Using cephalometric data, Ozbeck and colleagues[105] found a higher resting tongue posture in children following RME. Changes in tongue posture were not associated with respiratory disturbances and were noted to be stable after 24 months.[105] However, a systematic review noted that CBCT head and tongue position standardization is needed before drawing meaningful conclusions.[98]

Influence on mandibular positioning and growth

The ideal position of the mandible during maximum intercuspation is a subject of much debate. The shifting of the mandible to an anterior position has been proposed by some as a mechanism for an improved airway dynamics and jaw function.[106] Others follow orthopedic principles and favor a musculoskeletally stable mandibular position in which the mandibular condyles are in the most superior anterior position, resting against the posterior slopes of the articular eminences with the discs properly interposed.[107]

RME increases vertical dimension as occlusal contacts shift from fossae to cuspal inclines. RME has been hypothesized to lead to a "functional appliance–like effect" producing an anteriorly positioned mandible. Data suggest improvements in OSA following RME are not related to changes in mandibular positioning in class II patients.[108] Moreover, a study by Fastuca and colleagues[109] found improved AHI following RME but no significant difference in mandibular positioning. Conversely, Melgaco and colleagues[110] found a tendency for bilateral anterior and inferior condylar displacement following RME in a sample of patients with class I malocclusion without posterior crossbites.

Genetic and epigenetic influences ultimately drive mandibular growth and development.[77] Early management of a class II malocclusion may also have favorable results on the airway of a growing patient. Growth may be unpredictable; however, early orthodontic intervention can have a positive effect on both airway and facial symmetry.

Timing of treatment

Because fusion of the mid palatal suture occurs around puberty, late deciduous or early transitional dentition is an ideal time for RME.[111] Some suggest chronologic age is not reliable predictor of suture patency after age 11 years.[112] Treatment normally occurs before the patient has reached adult dentition; however, many studies include patients who are between the ages of 6 and 7.[91] Villa and others[113] concluded that orthodontic treatment should be initiated as soon as symptoms appear.

Benefits and risks of rapid maxillary expansion

The reported side-effect profile of RME is minimal. RME activation produces discomfort but tends to decrease as expansion continues.[114] Although there is considerable variation between patients, bonded, banded, toothborne, and non–tooth-bone-borne expanders are generally well tolerated by the patients.[115,116] Activation protocol has been noted to relate to perceived pain. Not surprisingly, Baldini and colleagues[117] found activation protocols involving less daily expansion correlate to less perceived pain. Additional risks and benefits of RME are listed in **Table 3**.

RAPID MAXILLARY EXPANSION APPLIANCES

Maxillary expanders, also referred to as palatal expanders, are orthopedic appliances routinely used by orthodontists in growing children.[116] Expansion appliances contain a midline jackscrew that is activated with an expansion key. Dentoalveolar expansion and tipping of teeth are potential outcomes of RME.[116] The degree of sutural separation versus dentoalveolar expansion may be influenced by design selection[116]

Hass and Hyrax appliances are examples of fixed appliances that are banded to permanent maxillary molars, primary molars, premolars, or a combination. Hass appliances include an acrylic portion that distributes forces across the soft tissues. Hyrax appliances lack acrylic and are considered to be more hygienic but may be associated with tipping of teeth.[116] Bonded acrylic expansion appliances are cemented to the occlusal surfaces of the teeth and can be used

Table 3
Benefits and risks of rapid maxillary expansion

Benefits	Risk
Create additional arch space	Potential problems if patient has adequate spacing Caution with congenitally missing lateral incisors
Decrease congestion of erupting maxillary anterior teeth	Distal drifting of incisors could lead to transposition or ectopic eruption
Level the curve of Wilson	Caution with anterior open bite or open bite tendency because expansion tends to "open" bites
Broaden the smile	Broad smile may reveal posterior restorations
Correct posterior crossbite	Potential to create "scissor bite" or buccal crossbite
Correct existing transverse deficiency	Potential to overexpand and negatively impact future orthognathic surgical treatment planning
Improve position of teeth in dental arch	May result in bony dehiscence, fenestrations, or displacement of teeth from alveolus
Controlled expansion with activation key	Patient may swallow or aspirate activation key or other component of expander
Parent responsible for activation of appliance	Miscommunication may lead to excessive or inadequate expansion
Fixed appliance	Possible need for recementation
Banded appliance	Possibility for dental caries or decalcification
Removable appliances	Appliances may become warped, misplaced
Speech changes are short term	Concern if patient undergoing speech therapy
Safe and well tolerated	Allergy to metal or acrylic possible
Minimally invasive	Some pain or discomfort possible Problematic for patients with profound gag reflex
Retention can be achieved with expansion device	Early removal may result in relapse Late removal may cause dental decalcification or soft tissue irritation
May decrease potential for future orthodontic/orthognathic treatment	May increase overall cumulative orthodontic treatment time

to intrude posterior teeth and control vertical dimensions.[116]

Treatment Technique

Records
Orthodontic records are recommended for treatment. Photos, diagnostic casts, panoramic radiographs, cephalometric radiographs, and tracings are examples of orthodontic records that may be obtained before and after RME therapy.

Bands and impressions
Proper band selection improves appliance retention. Ill-fitting bands may be associated with dislodgement of the final appliance. Orthodontic separators are typically placed between the teeth a few days before fitting and seating of orthodontic bands. Band options include plain bands and also bands with slots, tubes, or hooks used for orthodontic treatment. Bands with orthodontic attachments may be used if limited fixed appliances therapy is considered in conjunction with orthodontic expansion. Alignment and diastema closure are commonly performed together with RME therapy. Once appropriate bands are selected, a "pickup impression" can be obtained with a suitable impression material. If alginate is used, the impression should be poured in hard stone as early as possible to minimize distortion. The bands should be removed from the patient and secured in the impression. Cyanoacrylate, staples, or orthodontic wire may be used to stabilize the orthodontic bands before pouring of the impression. Some dental laboratories size and fit bands from the stone casts.

Seating the appliance
Separators are typically placed a few days before appliance cementation. Pumice may be used to clean the teeth before cementation. The appliance should fit without rocking. It may be helpful to apply composite resin to the palatal surfaces of the teeth to prevent the wire from migrating toward the occlusal surfaces during expansion.

Expansion and retention

Parents are provided a prescribed schedule for turning the jackscrew depending on the degree of expansion desired. Expansion can occur relatively quickly over a few weeks or can occur gradually over a period of months. Each quarter turn expands the appliance laterally approximately 0.25 mm. The key is turned until the next hole becomes visible. The patient may feel pressure in the anchoring teeth or nasal region during appliance activation.

Rapid expansion is considered 0.5 mm/d (two-quarter turns), whereas semi-rapid expansion is 0.25 mm/d (one-quarter turn).[77,118] Slow expansion protocol involves 0.5 to 1 mm/wk and results in minimal suture disruption. Data indicate long-term results are equivalent with each approach. Proffit and colleagues[77] recommends against using a rapid approach in preschool children because of the potential to cause adverse nasal changes. In adolescent patients, the rapid protocol may be used for 2 to 3 days to attempt to open the suture.[77] The presence of a diastema between the permanent maxillary incisors indicates opening of the midpalatal suture (**Fig. 2**).

Some relapse is expected; therefore, overcorrection is common when correcting a posterior crossbite. Ideal expansion is achieved when the palatal cusp of the upper molars is in contact with the lingual inclines of the buccal cusps of the mandibular molars.[116]

Retention

Retention may be achieved by leaving the original appliance in place for the desired time frame of 3 to 12 months. A less bulky fixed appliance, such as a transpalatal arch or Nance may also be used. Alternatively, a removable appliance such as a Hawley retainer may be considered for retention.

Additional Considerations

Bimaxillary (mandibulomaxillary) expansion

A bimaxillary expansion technique was performed in 45 children.[119] Fixed expansion appliances were used in both the maxillary and mandibular arches. Most of the patients demonstrated an improvement in sleep scores and symptoms; however, AHI worsened in a subset of patients.[119] Patients with retrognathia, mild OSA, small MP-SN, or counterclockwise mandibular growth worsened following expansion.[119]

Rapid maxillary expansion and mandibular advancement devices

Galeotti and colleagues[120] described a case of fixed maxillary expansion with simultaneous nighttime use of an MAD in a young child with OSA. Subjective improvement in symptoms were noted along with PSG-confirmed resolution of OSA.[120]

Rapid maxillary expansion and nocturnal enuresis

Orthodontic RME has been purposed as an option for treating children with NE who are resistant to medical therapy.[121] Clearly, more studies are needed to identify the role of orthodontic expansion in NE, and the placebo effect is considered to be high.[122] However, small studies have demonstrated a positive effect.[123] The spontaneous cure rate of NE is reported to be approximately 15%. A systematic review of RME for NE demonstrated a 31% cure rate.[124] A study by Al-Taai and colleagues[125] found plasma osmolality changes related to antidiuretic hormone with RME use. This preliminary work indicates a potential mechanism for RME as a treatment option for NE. Pediatricians or urologists should be included in any planned alternative treatment considerations for NE. RME may be part of a low-risk, multidisciplinary approach for some patients with recalcitrant NE.

Comprehensive orthodontic treatment

Before initiating RME, patients should ideally receive an orthodontic evaluation and treatment plan. Treatment of coexisting malocclusion is often performed in conjunction with expansion (**Fig. 3**).

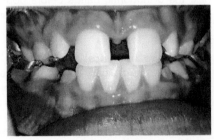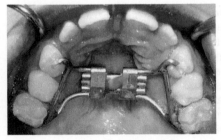

Fig. 2. Note the diastema between maxillary central incisors following expansion. The expansion screw may be blocked with resin to prevent additional activation.

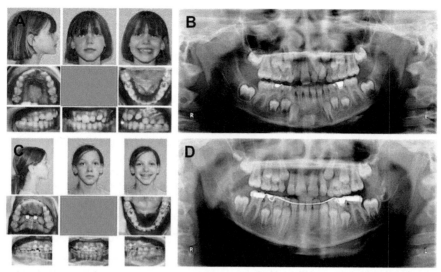

Fig. 3. (*A*) Patient with narrow palate, unilateral crossbite, and functional mandibular shift. Note the facial asymmetry. (*B*) Pretreatment panoramic radiograph demonstrating overretained left maxillary primary central incisor and ectopic eruption pathway of left permanent maxillary central incisor. (*C*) Progress photos demonstrating correction of posterior crossbite, widening of the palate, and improved facial symmetry. (*D*) Final panoramic radiograph after removal of rapid palatal expander and brackets. (*Courtesy of* Robert N. Galbreath DDS, MS, Virginia Beach, VA.)

Premolar extractions

Orthodontic treatment in a crowded mixed or adult dentition may involve extractions. A study by Larsen and colleagues[126] demonstrated that patients requiring premolar extractions are not at an increased risk of developing OSA. Moreover, a systematic review found insufficient data to conclude that extractions should be avoided.[127] In fact, some data suggest mesial movement of molars following extractions increased airway volume.[127] Conversely, Guilleminault and colleagues[128] analyzed pediatric patients with anodontia along with a small sample with history of orthodontic extractions and concluded that these patients may develop OSA at a later age due to decreased size of the oral cavity.

Multidisciplinary and Interdisciplinary Approach

Because of the complex nature of OSA, a multidisciplinary approach may optimize treatment. Although physicians are front-line providers, dental professionals, speech pathologists, nutritionists, and other health care providers can provide support.[129] An integrated approach should be considered.[113,129] Educating health care providers about the potential benefits of RME is an important step in interdisciplinary care. Patients with sleep-related concerns may see multiple medical specialists, including sleep physicians, otolaryngologists, pediatricians, neurologists, cardiologists, endocrinologists, psychiatrists, urologists, and pulmonologists. Oral and maxillofacial surgeons, orthodontists, pediatric dentists, and general dentists can provide unique options, including RME, MADs, and orthognathic surgery.

SUMMARY

Pediatric OSA is a serious medical condition with numerous health consequences. Dentists are well suited to recognize and provide medical referrals for pediatric patients at risk for OSA. Timely dental sleep medicine interventions may improve signs and symptoms of OSA in growing children. Data indicate that orthodontic and dentofacial orthopedic treatment may decrease obstructive respiratory events in some pediatric patients with OSA. Palatal expansion may be part of a comprehensive orthodontic treatment plan to correct a malocclusion and treat OSA. Orthognathic surgery, MADs, and oropharyngeal exercises also may have a role in the management of OSA in pediatric and adolescent patients.

REFERENCES

1. American Academy of Pediatrics. Clinical practice guideline on the diagnosis and management of childhood obstructive sleep apnea syndrome. Pediatrics 2012;130(3):576–684.

2. Alsubie HS, BaHammam SB. Obstructive sleep apnoea: children are not little adults. Paediatr Respir Rev 2017;21:72–9.

3. Ramar K, Dort LC, Katz SG, et al. Clinical practice guideline for the treatment of obstructive sleep apnea and snoring with oral appliance therapy: an update for 2015 an American Academy of Sleep Medicine and American Academy of dental sleep medicine clinical practice guideline. J Clin Sleep Med 2015;11(7):773–827.

4. American Academy of Pediatric Dentistry. Oral health policy on obstructive sleep apnea. Pediatr Dent 2017;39(6):96–8.

5. Leibovitz S, Haviv Y, Sharav Y, et al. Pediatric sleep-disordered breathing: role of the dentist. Quintessence Int 2017;48(8):639–45.

6. American Academy of Sleep Medicine. International classification of sleep disorders. 3rd edition. Darien (IL): American Academy of Sleep Medicine; 2014.

7. Huang YS, Guilleminault C. Pediatric obstructive sleep apnea: where do we stand? Adv Otorhinolaryngol 2017;80:136–44.

8. Blechner A, Williamson A. Consequences of OSA in children. Curr Probl Pediatr Adolesc Health Care 2016;46(1):19–26.

9. Bhattacharjii R, Kim J, Kherirandish-Gozal L, et al. Obesity and OSAS in children: a tale of inflammatory cascades. Pediatr Pulmonol 2011;4(6):313–23.

10. Ward JP, McMurtry IF. Mechanisms of hypoxic pulmonary vasoconstriction and their roles in pulmonary hypertension: new findings for an old problem. Curr Opin Pharmacol 2009;9(3):287–96.

11. Lee PC, Hwang B, Soong WJ, et al. The specific characteristics in children with obstructive sleep apnea and cor pulmonale. ScientificWorldJournal 2012;2012:757283.

12. Marcus CL, Greene MG, Carroll JL. Blood pressure in children with obstructive sleep apnea. Am J Respir Crit Care Med 1998;157(4 Pt 1):1098–103.

13. Nieminen P, Lopponen T, Tolonen U, et al. Growth and biochemical markers of growth in children with snoring and obstructive sleep apnea. Pediatrics 2002;109(4):e55.

14. Bar A, Tarasiuk A, Segev Y, et al. The effect of adenotonsillectomy on serum insulin-like growth factor-I and growth in children with obstructive sleep apnea syndrome. J Pediatr 1999;135(1):76–80.

15. Ahlqvist-Rastad J, Hultcrantz E, Melander H, et al. Body growth in relation to tonsillar enlargement and tonsillectomy. Int J Pediatr Otorhinolaryngol 1992;24(1):55–61.

16. Everett AD, Koch WC, Saulsbury FT. Failure to thrive due to obstructive sleep apnea. Clin Pediatr (Phila) 1987;26(2):90–2.

17. Marcus CL, Carroll JL, Koerner CB, et al. Determinants of growth in children with the obstructive sleep apnea syndrome. J Pediatr 1994;125(4):556–62.

18. Arens R, Muzumdar H. Childhood obesity and obstructive sleep apnea syndrome. J Appl Physiol (1985) 2010;108(2):436–44.

19. Rosen CL, Storfer-Isser A, Taylor HG, et al. Increased behavioral morbidity in school-aged children with sleep-disordered breathing. Pediatrics 2004;114(6):1640–8.

20. Kotagal S. A preschool-age child with obstructive sleep apnea. In: Olson EJ, Winkelman JW, editors. For the American Academy of Sleep Medicine, case book of sleep medicine. 2nd edition. Darien (IL): American Academy of Sleep Medicine; 2015. p. 149–53.

21. Gozal D. Sleep-disordered breathing and school performance in children. Pediatrics 1998;102(3 Pt1):616–20.

22. Ali NJ, Pitson D, Stradling JR. Natural history of snoring and related behaviour problems between the ages of 4 and 7 years. Arch Dis Child 1994;71(1):74–6.

23. Gislason T, Benediktsdottir B. Snoring, apneic episodes, and nocturnal hypoxemia among children 6 months to 6 years old. An epidemiologic study of lower limit of prevalence. Chest 1995;107(4):963–6.

24. Lumeng JC, Chervin RD. Epidemiology of pediatric obstructive sleep apnea. Proc Am Thorac Soc 2008;5(2):242–52.

25. Spilsbury JC, Storfer-Isser A, Kirchner HL, et al. Neighborhood disadvantage as a risk factor for pediatric obstructive sleep apnea. J Pediatr 2006;149:342–7.

26. Sanchez-Armengol A, Ruiz-Garcia A, Carmona-Bernal C, et al. Clinical and polygraphic evolution of sleep-related breathing disorders in adolescents. Eur Respir J 2008;32:1016–22.

27. Goldstein NA. Evaluation and management of pediatric obstructive sleep apnea Cummings Otolaryngology. 6th edition. Philidelphia: Saunders; 2015. p. 2855.

28. Mindell JA, Owens JA, Carskadon MA. Developmental features of sleep. Child Adolesc Psychiatr Clin N Am 1999;8:695–725.

29. Wooten CT, Shott SR. Evolving therapies to treat retroglossal and base-of-tongue obstruction in pediatric obstructive sleep apnea. Arch Otolaryngol Head Neck Surg 2010;136(10):983–7.

30. Torre C, Camacho M, Liu SY, et al. Epiglottis collapse in adult OSA: a systematic review. Laryngoscope 2016;126:1246–55.

31. Leonardis RL, Robison JG, Otteson TD. Evaluating the management of obstructive sleep apnea in

neonates and infants. JAMA Otolaryngol Head Neck Surg 2013;139(2):139–46.

32. Park JS, Chan DK, Parikh SR, et al. Surgical outcomes and sleep endoscopy for children with sleep-disordered breathing and hypotonia. Int J Pediatr Otorhinolaryngol 2016;90:99–106.

33. Floris-Mir, C Korayem M, Heo G, et al. Craniofacial morphological characteristics in children with obstructive sleep apnea syndrome: a systematic review and meta-analysis. J Am Dent Assoc 2013; 144(3):269–77. Available at: http://jada.ada.org.

34. Spilsbury JC, Storfer-Isser A, Rosen CL, et al. Remission and incidence of obstructive sleep apnea from middle childhood to late adolescence. Sleep 2015;38(1):23–9.

35. Guilleminault C, Akhtar F. Pediatric sleep-disordered breathing: new evidence on its development. Sleep Med Rev 2015;24:46–56.

36. Rosen CL, Larkin EK, Kirchner HL, et al. Prevalence and risk factors for sleep-disordered breathing in 8- to 11-year-old children: association with race and prematurity. J Pediatr 2003;142:383–9.

37. Redline SS, Tishler PV, Schluchter M, et al. Risk factors for sleep-disordered breathing in children: associations with obesity, race, and respiratory problems. Am J Respir Crit Care Med 1999;159: 1527–32.

38. Constantin E, Low NC, Dugas E, et al. Association between childhood sleep-disordered breathing and disruptive behavior disorders in childhood and adolescence. Behav Sleep Med 2015;13(6): 442–54.

39. Agarwal L, Tandon R, Kulshrestha R, et al. Adenoid faces and its management: an orthodontic perspective. Indian Journal of Orthodotics and Dentofacial Research 2016;(2):50–5.

40. Alexopoulos EI, Malakasioti G, Varlami V, et al. Nocturnal enuresis is associated with moderate-to-severe obstructive sleep apnea in children with snoring. Pediatr Res 2014;76(6):555–9.

41. Ferreira NM, Dos Santos JF, Dos Santos MB, et al. Sleep bruxism associated with obstructive sleep apnea in children. Cranio 2014;33(4):2015.

42. Lin CH, Guilleminault C. Current hypopnea scoring criteria underscore pediatric sleep disordered breathing. Sleep Med 2011;12(7):720–9.

43. Griebel ML. Sleep related breathing disorders in a child with achondroplasia. In: Olson EJ, Winkelman JW, editors. For the American Academy of Sleep Medicine, case book of sleep medicine. 2nd edition. Darien (IL): American Academy of Sleep Medicine; 2015.

44. Keating J, Park JH. Evaluation of current screening and treatment patterns for pediatric obstructive sleep apnea among practicing pediatric dentists in the United States: a pilot study. Pediatr Dent 2016;38(5):393–7.

45. Owens JA, Dalzell V. The use of BEARS sleep screening tool in a pediatric residents' community clinic. A pilot study. Sleep Med 2005;6(1): 63–9.

46. Chervin RD, Weatherly RA, Garetz SL, et al. Pediatric sleep questionnaire. Prediction of sleep apnea and outcomes. Arch Otolaryngol Head Neck Surg 2007;133:216–22.

47. Grunwell JR, McCracken C, Fortenberry J, et al. Risk factors leading to failed procedural sedation in children outside the operating room. Pediatr Emerg Care 2014;30(6):381–7.

48. Camacho M, Moller MW, Zaghi S, et al. Tongue-lip adhesion and tongue repositioning for obstructive sleep apnoea in Pierre Robin Sequence: a systematic review and meta-analysis. J Laryngol Otol 2017;131(5):378–83.

49. Rivero A, Durr M. Lingual tonsillectomy for pediatric persistent obstructive sleep apnea: a systematic review and meta-analysis. Otolaryngol Head Neck Surg 2017;157(6):940–7.

50. Redline S, Amin R, Bebee D, et al. The Childhood Adenotonsillectomy Trial (CHAT): rationale, design, and challenges of a randomized controlled trial evaluating a standard surgical procedure in a pediatric population. Sleep 2011;34(11):1509–17.

51. Marcus CL, Moore RH, Rosen CL, et al. A randomized trial of adenotonsillectomy for childhood sleep apnea. N Engl J Med 2013;368(25): 2366–76.

52. Taylor HR, Bowen SR, Beebe DW, et al. Cognitive effects of adenotonsillectomy for obstructive sleep apnea. Pediatrics 2016;138(2) [pii:e20154458].

53. Friedman M, Wilson M, Lin HC, et al. Updated systematic review of tonsillectomy and adenoidectomy for treatment of pediatric obstructive sleep apnea/hypopnea syndrome. Otolaryngol Head Neck Surg 2009;140(6):800–8.

54. Imanguli M, Ulualp SO. Risk factors for residual obstructive sleep apnea after adenotonsillectomy in children. Laryngoscope 2016;126(11):2624–9.

55. Bell RB, Turvey TA. Skeletal advancement for the treatment of obstructive sleep apnea in children. Cleft Palate Craniofac J 2001;38(2):147–54.

56. Miloro M. Mandibular distraction osteogenesis for pediatric airway management. J Oral Maxillofac Surg 2010;68(7):1512–23.

57. Conley RS. Orthodontic considerations related to sleep-disordered breathing. Sleep Med Clin 2010; 5:71–89.

58. Jackson GW. Orthodontic and orthognathic surgical treatment of a pediatric OSA patient. Case Rep Dent 2016;2016:5473580.

59. Dergin G, Aktop S, Varol A, et al. Complications related to surgically assisted rapid palatal expansion. Oral Surg Oral Med Oral Pathol Oral Radiol 2015;119(6):601–7.

60. Pomeranzt J. Management of persistent obstructive sleep apnea after adenotonsillectomy. Pediatr Ann 2016;45(5):e180–3.

61. Hawkins SW, Jensen EL, Simon SL, et al. Correlates of pediatric CPAP adherence. J Clin Sleep Med 2016;12(6):879–84.

62. Uong EC, Epperson M, Bathon SA, et al. Adherence to nasal positive airway pressure therapy among school-aged children and adolescents with obstructive sleep apnea syndrome. Pediatrics 2007;120(5):1203–11.

63. Roberts SD, Kapadia H, Greenlee G, et al. Midfacial and dental changes associated with nasal positive airway pressure in children with OSA and craniofacial conditions. J Clin Sleep Med 2016; 12(4):469–75.

64. Chan CC, Au CT, Lam HS, et al. Intranasal corticosteroids for mild childhood obstructive sleep apnea—a randomized, placebo-controlled study. Sleep Med 2015;16(3):358–63.

65. Kheirandish-Gozal D. Intranasal budesonide treatment for children with mild obstructive sleep apnea syndrome. Pedatrics 2008;122(1):e149–55.

66. Goldbart AD, Greenberg-Dolan S, Tai A. Montelukast for children with obstructive sleep apnea: a double-blind, placebo-controlled study. Pediatrics 2012;130(3):e575–80.

67. Kheirandish-Gozal D, Bandla HP, Gozal D. Monetlukast for children with obstructive sleep apnea: results of a double-blind, randomized, placebo-controlled trial. Ann Am Thorac Soc 2016;13(10): 1736–41.

68. Moeller JL, Coceani Paskay L, Gelb ML. Myofunctional therapy a novel treatment of pediatric sleep-disordered breathing. Sleep Med Clin 2014;9: 235–43.

69. Villa MP, Evangelisti M, Martella S, et al. Can myofunctional therapy increase tongue tone and reduce symptoms in children with sleep-disordered breathing? Sleep Breath 2017;21(4):1025–32.

70. Lione R, Franhi L, Huanca G, et al. Palatal surface volume in mouth breathing subjects evaluated with 3D analysis of digital dental casts: a controlled study. Eur J Orthod 2015;37:101–4.

71. Rossi RC, Rossi NJ, Carrieri Rossi MJ, et al. Dentofacial characteristics of oral breathers in different ages: a retrospective case-control study. Prog Orthod 2015;16:23.

72. Guilleminault C, Huang YS. From oral facial dysfunction to dysmorphism and the onset of pediatric OSA. Sleep Med Rev 2018;40:203–14.

73. Camacho M, Certal V, Abdullatif J, et al. Myofunctional therapy to treat obstructive sleep apnea: a systematic review and meta-analysis. Sleep 2015; 38(5):669–75.

74. Xiang M, Hu B, Liu Y, et al. Changes in airway dimensions following functional appliances in growing patients with skeletal class II malocclusion: a systematic review and meta-analysis. Int J Pediatr Otorhinolaryngol 2017;97:170–80.

75. Iwasaki T, Takemoto Y, Inada E, et al. Three-dimensional cone-beam computed tomography analysis of enlargement of the pharyngeal airway by the Herbst appliance. Am J Orthod Dentofacial Orthop 2014;146(6):776–85.

76. Carvalho FR, Lentini-Oliveira DA, Prado LB, et al. Oral appliances and functional orthopaedic appliances for obstructive sleep apnoea in children. Cochrane Database Syst Rev 2016;10: CD005520.

77. Proffit WR, Fields HW, Sarver DM. Contemporary orthodontics. 5th edition. Maryland Heights, MS: Elsevier Health Science. Mosby; 2014. p. 228–30.

78. O'Brien K, Wright J, Conboy F, et al. Early treatment for Class II division 1 malocclusion with the twin-block appliance. Am J Orthod Dentofacial Orthop 2009;135:573–9.

79. Idris G, Galland B, Robertson CJ, et al. Mandibular advancement appliances for sleep disordered breathing in children: a randomized crossover clinical trial. J Dent 2018;71:9–17.

80. Nazarali N, Altalibi M, Nazarali S, et al. Mandibular advancement appliances for the treatment of paediatric obstructive sleep apnea: a systematic review. Eur J Orthod 2015;37(6):618–26.

81. American Academy of Pediatric Dentistry. Guideline on management of the developing dentition and occlusion in pediatric dentistry. Pediatr Dent 2017;39(6):289–301.

82. McNamara JA, Lione R, Franchi L, et al. The role of rapid maxillary expansion in the promotion of oral and general health. Prog Orthod 2015;16:33.

83. Kiliaridis S, Mahboubi PH, Raadsheer MC, et al. Ultrasonographic thickness of the masseter muscle in growing individuals with unilateral crossbite. Angle Orthod 2007;77:607–11.

84. Kilic N, Kiki A, Oktay H. Condylar asymmetry in unilateral posterior crossbite patients. Am J Orthod Dentofacial Orthop 2008;133(3):382–7.

85. Villa MP, Castaldo R, Miano S, et al. Adenotonsillectomy and orthodontic therapy in pediatric obstructive sleep apnea. Sleep Breath 2014; 18(3):533–9.

86. Cistulli PA, Palmisano RG, Poole MD. Treatment of obstructive sleep apnea syndrome by rapid maxillary expansion. Sleep 1998;21(8):831–5.

87. Villa MP, Malagola C, Pagani J, et al. Rapid maxillary expansion in children with obstructive sleep apnea syndrome: 12-month follow-up. Sleep Med 2007;8128–34.

88. Villa MP, Rizzoli A, Miamo S, et al. Efficacy of rapid maxillary expansion in children with obstructive sleep apnea syndrome: 36 month follow-up. Sleep Breath 2011;15:179–84.

89. Buccheri A, Chine F, Fratto G, et al. Rapid maxillary expansion in obstructive sleep apnea in young patients: cardio-respiratory monitoring. J Clin Pediatr Dent 2017;41(4):312–6.

90. Vale F, Albergaria M, Carrilho E, et al. Efficacy of rapid maxillary expansion in the treatment of obstructive sleep apnea syndrome: a systematic review with meta-analysis. J Evid Based Dent Pract 2017;17(3):159–68.

91. Camacho M, Chang ET, Song SA, et al. Rapid maxillary expansion for pediatric obstructive sleep apnea: a systematic review and meta-analysis. Laryngoscope 2016;127:1712–9.

92. Pirelli P, Saponara M, Guilleminault C. Rapid maxillary expansion (RME) for pediatric obstructive sleep apnea: a 12-year follow-up. Sleep Med 2015;16(8):933–5.

93. Chervin RD, Ellenberg SS, Xiaoling H, et al. Prognosis for spontaneous resolution of OSA in children. Chest 2015;148(5):1204–13.

94. Iwasaki T, Saitoh I, Takemoto Y, et al. Improvement of nasal ventilation after rapid maxillary expansion evaluated with computational fluid dynamics. Am J Orthod Dentofacial Orthop 2012;141:269–78.

95. Oliveira De Felippe NL, Da Silveira AC, Viana G, et al. Relationship between rapid maxillary expansion and nasal cavity size and airway resistance: short- and long-term effects. Am J Orthod Dentofacial Orthop 2008;134(3):370–82.

96. Iwasaki T, Saitoh I, Takemoto Y, et al. Tongue posture improvement and pharyngeal airway enlargement as secondary effects of rapid maxillary expansion: a cone-beam computed tomography study. Am J Orthod Dentofacial Orthop 2013; 143(2):235–45.

97. Fastuca R, Perinetti G, Zecca PA, et al. Airway compartments volume and oxygen saturation changes after rapid maxillary expansion: a longitudinal correlation study. Angle Orthod 2015;85(6): 955–61.

98. Di Carlo G, Saccucci M, Ierardo G, et al. Rapid maxillary expansion and upper airway morphology: a systematic review on the role of cone beam computed tomography. Biomed Res Int 2017; 2017:5460429.

99. American Academy of Pediatric Dentistry. Guideline on prescribing dental radiographs for infants, children, adolescents, and persons with special health care needs. Pediatr Dent 2017;39(6):319–21.

100. Di Vece L, Doldo T, Faleri G, et al. Rhinofibroscopic and rhinomanometric evaluation of patients with maxillary contraction treated with rapid maxillary expansion. A prospective pilot study. J Clin Pediatr Dent 2018;42(1):27–31.

101. Wang de Y, Lee HP, Bruce R, et al. Impacts of fluid dynamics simulation in study of nasal airflow physiology and pathophysiology in realistic human three-dimensional nose models. Clin Exp Otorhinolaryngol 2012;5(4):181–7.

102. Zhao Y, Nguyen M, Gohl E, et al. Oropharyngeal airway changes after rapid palatal expansion evaluated with cone-beam computed tomography. Am J Orthod Dentofacial Orthop 2010;137:S71–8.

103. El H, Palomo JM. Three-dimensional evaluation of upper airway following rapid maxillary expansion. Angle Orthod 2014;84(2):265–73.

104. Fastuca R, Meneghel M, Zecca PA, et al. Multimodal airway evaluation in growing patients after rapid maxillary expansion. Eur J Paediatr Dent 2015;16(2):129–34.

105. Ozbeck MM, Memikoglu UT, Altug-Atac AT, et al. Stability of maxillary expansion and tongue posture. Angle Orthod 2009;79(2):214–20.

106. Gelb ML. Airway centric TMJ philosophy. J Calif Dent Assoc 2014;42(8):551–62 [discussion: 560–2].

107. Okeson JP. Evolution of occlusion and temporomandibular disorder in orthodontics: past, present, and future. Am J Orthod Dentofacial Orthop 2015; 147(5):S216–23.

108. Lione R, Brunelli V, Franchi L, et al. Mandibular response after rapid maxillary expansion in class II growing patients: a pilot randomized controlled trial. Prog Orthod 2017;18(1):36.

109. Fastuca R, Zecca PA, Caprioglio A. Role of mandibular displacement and airway size in improving breathing after rapid maxillary expansion. Prog Orthod 2014;15:40.

110. Melgaco CA, Columbano NJ, Jurach EM, et al. Immediate changes in condylar position after rapid maxillary expansion. Am J Orthod Dentofacial Orthop 2014;145(6):771–9.

111. Monini S, Malagola C, Villa MP, et al. Rapid maxillary expansion for the treatment of nasal obstruction in children younger than 12 years. Arch Otolaryngol Head Neck Surg 2009;135(1):22–7.

112. Angelieri F, Cevidanes LHS, Franchi L, et al. Midpalatal suture maturation: classification method for individual assessment before rapid maxillary expansion. Am J Orthod Dentofacial Orthop 2013;144(5):759–69.

113. Villa MP, Rizolli A, Rabasco J, et al. Rapid maxillary expansion outcomes in treatment of OSA in children. Sleep Med 2015;16(6):709–16.

114. Halicioglu K, Kiki A, Yavus I. Subjective symptoms of RME patients treated with three different screw activation protocols: a randomised clinical trial. Aust Orthod J 2012;28(2):225–31.

115. Feldman I, Bazargani F. Pain and discomfort during the first week of rapid maxillary expansion (RME) using two different RME appliances: a randomized controlled trial. Angle Orthod 2017;87(3):391–6.

116. McNamara JA, Brudon WL. Orthodontics and dentofacial orthopedics. Ann Arbor (MI): Needham Press, Inc; 2001. p. 211–31.

117. Baldini A, Nota A, Santariello C, et al. Influence of activation protocol on perceived pain during rapid maxillary expansion. Angle Orthod 2015;85(6): 1015–20.

118. Hoxha S, Kaya-Sezginer E, Bakar-Ates F, et al. Effect of semi-rapid maxillary expansion in children with obstructive sleep apnea syndrome: 5-month follow-up study. Sleep Breath 2018. [Epub ahead of print].

119. Quo SD, Hyunh N, Guilleminault C. Bimaxillary expansion therapy for pediatric sleep-disordered breathing. Sleep Med 2017;30:45–51.

120. Galeotti A, Festa P, Pavone M, et al. Effects of simultaneous palatal expansion and mandibular advancement in a child suffering from OSA. Acta Otorhinolograyngol Ital 2016;36(4):328–32.

121. Schütz-Fransson U, Kurol J. Rapid maxillary expansion effects on nocturnal enuresis in children: a follow-up study. Angle Orthod 2008;78(2):201–8.

122. Oshagh M, Bahramnia F, Aminsharifi AR, et al. Effects of maxillary expansion and placebo effect of appliances on nocturnal enuresis—preliminary results. Cent European J Urol 2014;67(1):51–5.

123. Hyla-Kleot L, Truszel M, Paradysz A, et al. Influence of orthodontic rapid maxillary expansion on nocturnal enuresis in children. Biomed Res Int 2015;2015:201039.

124. Poorsattar-Bejeh Mir K, Poorsattar-Bejeh Mir A, Poorsattar-Bejeh Mir M, et al. Rapid palatal expansion to treat nocturnal enuretic children: a systematic review and meta-analysis. J Dent (Shiraz) 2015;16(3):138–48.

125. Al-Taai N, Alfatlawi F, Ransjö M, et al. Effect of rapid maxillary expansion on monosymptomatic primary nocturnal enuresis. Angle Orthod 2015;85(1): 102–8.

126. Larsen AJ, Rindal DB, Hatch JP, et al. Evidence supports no relationship between obstructive sleep apnea and premolar extraction: an electronic health records review. J Clin Sleep Med 2015; 11(12):1443–8.

127. Hu Z, Yin X, Liao J, et al. The effect of teeth extraction for orthodontic treatment on the upper airway: a systematic review. Sleep Breath 2015;19(2): 441–51.

128. Guilleminault C, Abad VC, Chiu HY, et al. Missing teeth and pediatric obstructive sleep apnea. Sleep Breath 2016;20(2):561–8.

129. Camacho M, Ryhn MJ, Fukui CS, et al. Multidisciplinary sleep clinic: a patient-centered approach. Cranio 2017;35(2):129.

Skeletal Surgery for Obstructive Sleep Apnea

José E. Barrera, MD[a,b,c],*

KEYWORDS

- Obstructive sleep apnea • Surgery success • Surgery technique • Skeletal surgery
- Hyoid myotomy and suspension • Genioglossal advancement • Sliding genioplasty
- Maxillomandibular advancement

KEY POINTS

- Combined with a uvulopalatopharyngoplasty, tongue-base surgeries, including the genioglossus advancement (GA), sliding genioplasty, and hyoid myotomy and suspension, have been developed to target hypopharyngeal obstruction.
- Total airway surgery consisting of maxillomandibular advancement with or without GA has shown significant success in patients with obstructive sleep apnea (OSA).
- Skeletal procedures for OSA with or without a palatal procedure is a proven technique for relieving airway obstruction during sleep.

INTRODUCTION

Obstructive sleep apnea (OSA) continues to be a pervasive condition that is linked to an increased incidence of cardiovascular diseases, endocrine disorders, and overall increased health care utilization.[1] Multilevel surgery has been established as the mainstay of treatment for the surgical management of OSA. Skeletal surgery for OSA has traditionally consisted of a phased protocol to address airway obstruction secondary to nasopharyngeal, oropharyngeal, and hypopharyngeal obstruction. Combined with a uvulopalatopharyngoplasty (UPPP), tongue-base surgeries, including the genioglossus advancement (GA), sliding genioplasty (SG), and hyoid myotomy and suspension, have been developed to target hypopharyngeal obstruction. Total airway surgery, consisting of maxillomandibular advancement (MMA) with or without GA, has shown significant success in patients with OSA.

Skeletal procedures for OSA with or without a palatal procedure are a proven technique for relieving airway obstruction during sleep.[2]

It has been well established that skeletal advancement procedures typically accomplish a goal of 8 to 14 mm of advancement, thus increasing tension on the pharyngeal, genioglossus, and geniohyoid muscles with the goal of reducing the severity of sleep apnea.[1,3,4] Patients are traditionally selected for surgery based on the level of obstruction, which often occurs at the level of the base of tongue, although most patients demonstrate retropalatal obstruction as well. Since the introduction of a skeletal surgery to advance the genioglossus muscle along with UPPP, as described by Riley and colleagues,[1] multilevel reconstruction surgery has demonstrated improved outcomes in relieving OSA in those who demonstrate multilevel obstruction.[3,4]

This article was previously published in volume 49, issue 6 (December 2016) of *Otolaryngologic Clinics of North America*.

There are no commercial interests nor conflicts of interest associated with this publication. There is no funding for this work.

[a] Department of Surgery, Uniformed Services University, Bethesda, MD, USA; [b] Department of Otolaryngology, University of Texas Health Sciences Center, San Antonio, TX, USA; [c] Texas Facial Plastic Surgery and ENT, 14603 Huebner Road, Building 1, San Antonio, TX 78209, USA

* Texas Facial Plastic Surgery and ENT, 555 East Basse Road, Suite 201, San Antonio, TX 78209.

E-mail address: admin@drjosebarrera.com

Sleep Med Clin 13 (2018) 549–558
https://doi.org/10.1016/j.jsmc.2018.07.006

Although physical examination, drug-induced sleep endoscopy (DISE), and polysomnography (PSG) help to guide the clinician's decision-making process in selecting patients who are candidates for GA, SG, or MMA combined with UPPP, intraoperative factors, such as length and width of the velum, degree of palatal and tongue-base obstruction, and concomitant lateral pharyngeal wall obstruction, are currently being studied. DISE[5,6] and sleep MRI[7,8] have emerged as modalities to diagnose the site of airway obstruction before surgery.

Preoperative Considerations

All patients considered for skeletal surgery are first diagnosed by PSG, Epworth evaluation, and fiberoptic laryngoscopy. Candidates for surgery present with an apnea-hypopnea index (AHI) of more than 5 events per hour, and/or a respiratory disturbance index (RDI) greater than 5 with an Epworth Sleepiness Scale (ESS) greater than 8, who either did not tolerate, or refused a trial of continuous positive airway pressure (PAP). Presurgical patients present with evidence of obstruction as demonstrated by awake physical examination documenting Friedman II or III classification. Exclusion criteria for skeletal surgery include age younger than 12 years, chronic pulmonary disease on oxygen, and those affected with an untreated sleep disorder other than OSA that represents their primary sleep disorder. Preoperative assessment included history taking; ESS evaluation; complete physical examination; and PSG. Outcomes are defined by success, cure, and responder criteria. Success is defined as an AHI less than 20 and/or a 50% decrease in AHI of the preoperative value. Cure is defined as an AHI less than 5 events per hour. Responder is defined as significant improvement in the AHI and/or RDI after surgical intervention.

Obstruction can occur at a number of points in the airway. Physical examination of these patients may reveal hypertrophy of the adenoids and tonsils, retrognathia, micrognathia, macroglossia, deviation of the nasal septum, turbinate hypertrophy, a thick short neck, or tumors in the nasopharynx or hypopharynx. Both primary and secondary medical conditions are associated with OSA, owing to their effects on the upper airway anatomy. These may include temporomandibular joint disorders, myxedema, goiter, acromegaly, and lymphoma.

Fiberoptic nasopharyngoscopy is used to identify obstruction at the nasopharynx, oropharynx, and hypopharynx, and to rule out laryngeal anomalies. It can help estimate the degree of lateral wall collapse, palatal narrowing, and tongue-base obstruction. The site of obstruction can be classified by Fujita classification, with type I being palatal obstruction only, type II presenting as a combined palatal and tongue-base obstruction, and type III a tongue-base obstruction pattern only. Without performing fiberoptic evaluation, the site of obstruction may not be discernable.

Cephalometric evaluation is a simple way to evaluate individual patient upper airway site of obstruction. Cephalometric evaluation has long been used in evaluation of the airway in OSA. The metrics used for evaluation are SNA, SNB, PNS, Mandibular angle, posterior airway space (PAS), and MP-H (**Fig. 1**). These metrics are used to evaluate preoperative obstruction and follow postoperative results. It is recommended that this 2-dimensional radiograph be supplemented with a 3-dimensional fiberoptic to evaluate the airway. At our institution, the most consistent finding is a narrowed PAS and low hyoid position (MP-H).[9]

The definitive objective test is a study during sleep. The gold standard at present is an attended PSG evaluation. This level I study assesses the cardiorespiratory system, revealing oxygenation information, and records electroencephalogram, electrooculogram, and electromyogram. It reveals sleep stage information and estimates the percentage of apnea, hypopneas, and respiratory-related events during sleep. Ambulatory studies are estimated as level III and do not determine sleep stage data.

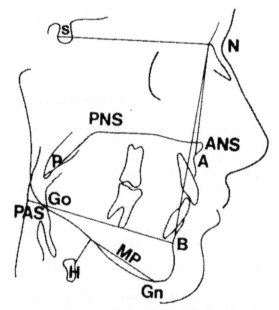

Fig. 1. Cephalometric figure. (*From* Riley RW, Powell NB, Guilleminault C. Inferior mandibular osteotomy and hyoid myotomy suspension for obstructive sleep apnea: a review of 55 patients. J Oral Maxillofac Surg 1989;47(2):160; with permission.)

Surgical Technique

Retropalatal obstruction is addressed with UPPP. Fujita and colleagues[10] introduced UPPP with tonsillectomy in 1979. Many modifications have been published; the basic procedure involves palate shortening with closure mucosal incisions, tonsillectomy, and lateral pharyngoplasty. For multilevel surgery candidates, patients undergo a UPPP with GA or SG.

Genioglossal Advancement

The GA must be distinguished from tongue suspension. The advancement of the geniotubercle in the GA procedure is distinct from suture fixation and suspension of the tongue base. The tongue suspension technique does not advance the mandible and is not considered a skeletal procedure. GA is performed as described by Riley and colleagues.[11] To review, after local anesthetic with a concentration of 1:100,000, epinephrine is injected at the lower gingivolabial sulcus, an incision is created along the anterior mandible. Subperiosteal dissection is then achieved exposing the anterior face of the mandible along its inferior border and then laterally identifying the mental neurovascular bundles. A horizontal window osteotomy is then created using a sagittal saw approximately 5 mm below the roots of the canine and approximately 10 mm above the inferior border of the mandible. The bone cut is then connected with 2 vertical osteotomies completing the rectangular window. Making a bicortical anterior osteotomy performs the GA. The width of the mandible, which had been pulled forward via the window osteotomy, is measured. The facial cortex and medullary bone is then removed and the lingual cortex holding the origin of the genioglossus muscle is rotated perpendicular to the window osteotomy. The osteotomized segment is then secured inferiorly with a single bicortical titanium screw. Closure is performed with a 3 to 0 chromic with closure of the mentalis muscle and gingiva-buccal sulcus.

Sliding Genioplasty Technique

The SG is an advancement genioplasty that is occasionally recommended for patients with microgenia due to both a retrognathic and foreshortened mandible. Patients in whom the GA cannot be performed due to increased risk for tooth injury or in patients with significant retrognathia greater than 2 cm from the subnasale vertical tangent may be considered for SG. The SG procedure seldom includes the entire genial tubercle, thereby not affecting pull on the genioglossal muscle. It will likely pull the geniohyoid muscle that may lead to

an unfavorable vector on the tongue base. The procedure may be amenable for patients with retroepiglottic obstruction. The SG is performed through subperiosteal dissection with exposure of the inferior border of the anterior mandible. A reciprocating saw is used to cut both lateral edges of the parasymphysis along its inferior border and then laterally tapering the cut below the mental neurovascular bundles. The SG operation is often performed for both functional and aesthetic concerns. When the anterior osteotomy incorporates the geniotubercle through adjacent vertical window osteotomies, the operation is described as a mortised genioplasty. A patient with mild OSA with microgenia and nasal obstruction is depicted with postoperative cure in OSA after functional rhinoplasty and SG in **Fig. 2**.

Hyoid Myotomy and Suspension

There are 2 generally accepted techniques in performing hyoid myotomy and suspension; the hyoid-mandibular and the hyoid-thyroid technique.[1,12,13] The author describes the hyoid-thyroid technique in this publication. The hyoid bone is a U-shaped bone suspended by the omohyoid, mylohyoid, and geniohyoid muscle; hyoepiglottic ligament; and accessory strap and laryngeal muscles. Its intimate connection with the tongue base and epiglottis makes it a viable technique for addressing hypopharyngeal obstruction. The hyoid-thyroid technique is performed through a cervical neck incision overlying the hyoid bone. Dissection is performed in a subplatysmal plane to expose the hyoid bone. Infrahyoid release of the strap muscles is performed using electrocautery medial to the greater cornu of the hyoid. Mobilization and suspension of the hyoid bone over the thyroid cartilage is performed using 2 to 0 Prolene sutures as depicted. The hyoid-thyroid technique may be performed under local anesthesia with fiberoptic evaluation of the hypopharynx or under general anesthesia with concomitant GA, SG, or UPPP.

Maxillomandibular Advancement

Patients who have had incomplete response or failed to respond to phase I intervention may be considered for a phase II operation or MMA. In addition, patients with significant skeletal-dental deformity with OSA may be candidates for MMA. The MMA advances the midface and provides more room for the tongue. Additionally, the sagittal split osteotomy of the mandible places additional tension on the tongue-hyoid complex. Several publications have described the use of MMA in treating large series of patients with OSA.[14–19]

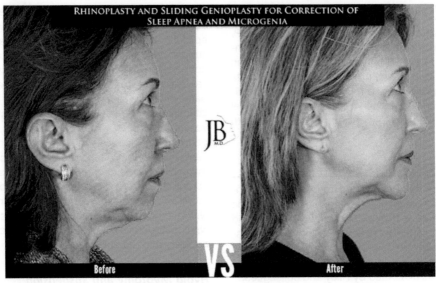

Fig. 2. SG patient with mild OSA (*left*: before; *right*: after functional rhinoplasty and SG).

A bilateral sagittal ramus osteotomy is performed through a posterior gingivo-buccal incision. Care is taken to identify the lingula of the mesial ascending ramus and the inferior alveolar nerve. A Hunsuck osteotomy is made with Lindeman burr or reciprocating blade (**Fig. 3**). The sagittal osteotomy then connects the ascending ramus cuts with the Dalpont osteotomy in the anterior mandible (**Fig. 4**). The ramus is then split with osteotomes. The amount of advancement is determined preoperatively from the orthognathic model surgery and/or virtual plan. Adjunctive orthodontic treatment is frequently necessary to obtain the desired occlusion and to eliminate dental compensations that would otherwise limit the amount of advancement. Presurgical orthodontic evaluation with modeling may be considered before surgery but is not necessary. A thorough discussion is made with the patient to

consider accompanying skeletal-dental abnormalities, and perioperative and postoperative management. Most patients retain their preoperative occlusion without need for orthodontic management. After advancement with the standard surgical technique, the fragments are rigidly fixed with screws or bone plates. For large advancements of 7 mm or more, long-term stability is enhanced with a 5-day to 7-day course of maxillomandibular fixation using orthodontic bands.

Combined advancement of the maxilla and mandible is the most recent and efficacious surgical procedure for the treatment of OSA. The surgical technique includes a standard Le Fort I osteotomy in combination with the aforementioned mandibular sagittal split osteotomy. A concomitant GA, as previously described, is an adjunct and recommended to improve tongue advancement (**Fig. 5**). MMA surgery may result

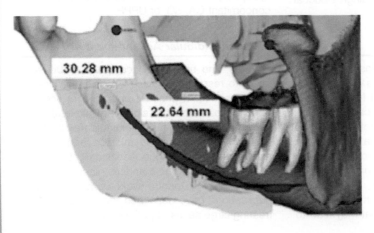

Fig. 3. MMA. Note Hunsuck osteotomy is made above the lingula. In this VSP, the width of the ramus at the osteotomy is 30.28 mm with the inferior alveolar nerve emanating 22.64 mm from the ramus. The inferior alveolar nerve is shown in red.

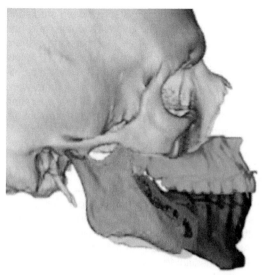

Fig. 4. MMA surgery depicting Lefort I osteotomy with bilateral sagittal split osteotomy with fixation is shown. Note sagittal split and anterior Dalpont osteotomy proposed and shown with advancement.

in some facial change, which is most often favorable. However, the patient must be made aware of the possibility of any unfavorable aesthetic outcomes that may occur from this surgical procedure.

MANDIBULAR SETBACK PROCEDURES

Mandibular setback procedures are composed of SG setbacks for a prominent chin in the aesthetic patients and bilateral sagittal split osteotomies performed for setback in the class III prognathic patients. In a small number of patients, a mandibular setback procedure can be the initiating factor in the development of OSA. Riley and colleagues[20] reported on 2 patients who developed OSA after mandibular setback surgery for correction of class III malocclusion and skeletal prognathism. Preoperative evaluation of these patients showed no symptoms of sleep apnea before surgery. Postoperatively, both patients began to snore loudly. PSG confirmed the presence of OSA syndrome. A comparative examination of the preoperative and postoperative lateral cephalograms of each patient showed a more inferiorly positioned hyoid bone and a narrowing of the pharyngeal airway. The report publication warns of the possibility of resultant OSA secondary to mandibular setback surgery, therefore caution should be heralded with this technique.

In an attempt to identify those patients potentially at risk for OSA, all patients who are planned for mandibular setback procedures should be questioned preoperatively and postoperatively about the presence or absence of snoring, excessive daytime sleepiness, or observed apneas during sleep. A PSG is recommended before consideration of mandibular setback procedures in these patients. Although the vast majority of patients who undergo mandibular setbacks are able to adapt to the changes in the skeletal and muscular apparatus, there is a subset of patients who may be at risk for developing overt signs of OSA.

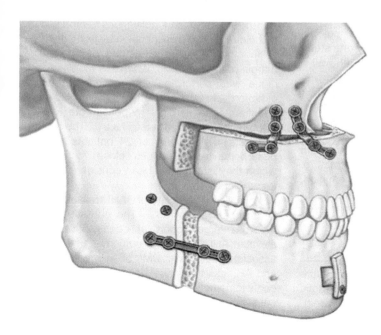

Fig. 5. MMA with GA. (*From* Barrera JE, Powell NB, Riley RW. Facial skeletal surgery in the management of adult obstructive sleep apnea syndrome. Clinics in Plastic Surgery 2007;34(3):565–73; with permission.)

SURGICAL RESULTS
Genioglossal Advancement

GA is a simple technique that does not move the teeth or jaw and therefore does not affect the dental bite. The GA is a procedure performed as a solitary hypopharyngeal procedure or in combination with MMA.[21] The technique places the genioglossus under tension and this tension may be sufficient to keep the base of tongue region open during sleep. This procedure does not gain more room for the tongue and thus must be considered a limited procedure that is dependent on the thickness of the individual's anterior mandible (mean thickness 12–18 mm). In addition, the existing laxity to the tongue during sleep is a factor on how much tension is gained when the genial tubercle is moved. In a flaccid tongue, the movement may all or partially be taken up by the advancement and little or no improvement may be attained. A paucity exists in determining the amount of tension needed or the critical distance the genial tubercle needs to move for effective posterior airway space improvement. An early study has determined that the tension-to-width ratio associated with geniotubercle advancement surgery may be an indicator for surgical response in patients with OSA.[22] These 2 factors limit our preoperative ability to accurately or consistently predict clinical outcomes. A meta-analysis evaluated success rates of genioglossal advancement to be between 39% and 78%.[23] Results of GA as a sole procedure for treatment of hypopharyngeal obstruction has been published in patients with severe OSA with success of more than 60% in 3 studies and oxyhemoglobin saturation results in 2 studies showing improvement in low oxyhemoglobin saturation (LSAT) in both studies. Only one study controlled for body mass index (BMI) and all 4 studies were level 4 Evidence based Medicine (EBM). The overall success rate was 62%. Our published clinical outcomes for success rates for GA with UPPP are 61%. Other centers have reported similar results with this procedure.

Complications associated with GA include tooth injury or loss, paresthesias, mandibular fracture, difficulty swallowing, wound infection, nonunion, and malunion of the mandible. Evaluation of swallow before and after GA has shown no increased incidence of swallow or speech dysfunction.[24]

Sliding Genioplasty

SG is considered a surgical adjunctive procedure mostly used in orthognathic surgery and aesthetic chin augmentation surgery. The mortised genioplasty technique described, which incorporates the genioglossus with an SG, has been studied in patients with OSA. The overall success rate has been reported to be 48%. In this study, there were 2 factors contributing to success: (1) a low preoperative BMI, BMI less than 30, and (2) a preoperative AHI less than 50. If these factors were ascribed, the successful result of the operation was 64% and 71%, respectively, in these subsets of patients.[25]

Genioglossal Advancement with Hyoid Myotomy

In 1989, Riley and colleagues[1,12] published a review of 55 patients with OSA who were treated with GA and hyoid myotomy with suspension (GAHM). Forty-two patients presented with type II Fujita classification showing obstruction at both the oropharynx and hypopharynx and received concomitant UPPP and GAHM. Six patients were determined to have obstruction localized to the base of the tongue (type III) and underwent GAHM only. Seven patients had failed previous UPPP and also underwent GAHM alone. All patients were reevaluated 6 months following surgery by PSG. Thirty-seven patients (67%) were considered to be responders to surgery based on the PSG results. GA ranged from 8 to 18 mm with a mean of 13 mm. All responders to surgery showed significant improvement in their RDI and oxygen desaturation events. Eighteen patients (33%) were considered nonresponders and failed to show significant improvement by PSG. The presence of preexisting chronic obstructive pulmonary disease was found to be a determining factor in increasing the risk of failure.

In 1994, Riley and colleagues[13] modified his technique for hyoid suspension by fixing the hyoid to the thyroid cartilage instead of the anterior margin of the mandible. When this modified technique was performed with inferior mandibular osteotomy, in lieu of the original hyoid suspension technique, the surgical response rate (with or without UPPP) was raised to 79.2%. The 5 nonresponders in this study of 24 patients achieved postoperative RDI values close to levels at which they would have been considered surgical responders.

A meta-analysis review of GAHM reveals an overall success rate of 55%. The published studies report a large cohort of obese patients with elevated AHI. Successful outcomes of 74% were associated with lower BMI, LSAT greater than 70, and AHI less than 60. A favorable SNB angle on cephalometric evaluation portended improved success rates.[23] Other investigators have reported that patients who have undergone GAHM have improved outcomes when presenting with normal pulmonary function, normal skeletal mandibular development, and the absence of obesity.[26] The most serious reported complication from a hyoid suspension has been severe aspiration in one patient, in which the thyrohyoid membrane was totally sectioned.[27] Other complications have included wound infections, transient sensory disturbances of the mental nerve, and mandibular fracture. An advantage to hyoid suspension is that it circumvents the need for maxillomandibular fixation and does not affect the occlusion.[26,27]

Hyoid Myotomy and Suspension

Success rates have varied in hyoid myotomy and suspension from 17% to 78% in 4 studies, all level 4 EBM.[23] However, these studies have been reported with associated UPPP or GA surgeries. In addition, the literature has not clearly delineated surgical results by hyoid suspension technique.

A recent meta-analysis evaluated tongue suspension with UPPP, GA with UPPP, and GA with tongue suspension and hyoid-to-mandibular suspension. The results demonstrated success in 62.3%, 61.6%, and 61.1%, respectively. There was no significant difference between groups 2 and 3 compared with group 1. However, when tongue suspension was performed alone, the success rate dropped to 36.6%.[28]

Maxillomandibular Advancement

Several investigators have described the use of MMA in treating large series of patients with OSA.[14–19,29,30] In a series of 23 patients, Waite and colleagues[14] reported surgical success with MMA as 65% based on a postsurgical RDI of less than 10. Riley and colleagues[15] reported the largest series of patients with OSA treated with MMA in which 98% (89 of 91) were successfully treated based on a postoperative RDI of less than 20 with at least a 50% reduction in the RDI compared with the preoperative study. Hochban and colleagues[16] reported a 98% success rate on 38 patients with OSA consecutively treated with a 10-mm MMA as the primary surgery with postoperative RDI less than 10 as the criteria to success. Prinsell[17] reported a 100% success rate based on a postoperative RDI of less than 15, an apnea index (AI) of less than 5, or a reduction in the RDI and AI of greater than 60% in patients who underwent MMA with and without GA. Lee and colleagues[18] proposed a 3-phased protocol for the surgical treatment of patients with OSA whereby phase I consisted of UPPP and GA or SG. If not successful, in phase 2, patients underwent MMA. A hyoid myotomy and suspension was reserved as a phase 3 surgery for failure. Phase 1 patients achieved success in 69% of cases (24 of 35 patients). Of the 11 stage 1 failures, 3 elected to proceed to phase 2 with MMA. All patients who underwent MMA had a postoperative RDI of less than 10, indicating a 100% response rate. No patient required hyoid myotomy and suspension. Bettega and colleagues[19] treated 51 consecutive patients with OSA, with 44 patients achieving a success rate of 22.7% (10 of 44) after UPPP and GAHM. Twenty patients underwent MMA as part of a phase 2 protocol. Of these, 75% (15 of 20) were considered to be surgical responders based on a postoperative RDI of less than 15 and at least a 50% reduction in the RDI. Of the 5 failures, 3 had postoperative RDIs of less than 20.

Riley and colleagues[29] describe MMA surgery as being a total airway surgery, having an effect on the posterior airway space (PAS) in the retropalatal and retrolingual space. PAS consistently increases with MMA. Caples and colleagues[30] published a meta-analysis comparing primary versus phased (secondary) MMA. In 234 patients receiving primary MMA, the mean preoperative AHI across all studies was 54.5 events per hour with resultant AHI of 7.7 events per hour postoperative. In 201 patients receiving secondary MMA, the mean preoperative AHI was 68.3 events per hour with 8.9 events per hour postoperatively. The mean BMI of patients with primary MMA was 29.1 compared with 36.6 in patients with secondary MMA. Holty and Guillenminault[31] published their meta-analysis reporting the clinical efficacy and safety of MMA surgery. Twenty-seven published articles reported on 320 patients with a mean AHI of 63.9 events per hour and a postoperative improvement of 9.5 events per hour postoperatively (P>.001). They reported that success was achieved with the greater degree of maxillary advancement. The major and minor complication rates were reported at 1.0% and 3.1%. Potential complications of MMA include surgical relapse, nonunion, bleeding, malocclusion, infection, unfavorable changes in facial appearance, and permanent or temporary sensory disturbances of the inferior alveolar and infraorbital nerves.[26] The long-term skeletal stability of MMA has been shown to be quite good. Louis and colleagues[32] showed a mean relapse of 0.9 ± 1.8 mm among 20 patients receiving maxillary advancement who underwent MMA for OSA with a mean follow-up period of 18.5 months (range 6–29 months). There was no statistical difference in the 3 groups based on advancement of 6 mm, 7 to 9 mm, and 10 mm or greater. Other reports have confirmed the stability of MMA surgery long term. Nimkarn and colleagues[33] showed that in 19 MMAs with SG patients that surgical stability was achieved over 1 year.[33]

MMA is considered the most efficacious procedure for expanding the pharyngeal airway and improving or eliminating OSA. It remains the best current alternative to tracheostomy.[26] Indications for this procedure include severe mandibular deficiency (SNB <74°), moderate to severe OSA (RDI >15, oxygen desaturations <90%), hypopharyngeal narrowing, and failure of other forms of treatment.[26] The success rate of MMA appears to increase when adjunctive procedures, such as UPPP, GA, lingual tonsillectomy and midline glossectomy, and nasal reconstruction, are considered in the phased treatment of patients with OSA.

Adjunctive orthodontic therapy may be considered in patients selected for MMA as long as airway protection by way of PAP therapy or an oral appliance as determined by PSG is ensured. Presurgical orthodontics improves the postoperative occlusion and eliminates preexisting dental compensations that would otherwise limit the amount of advancement. Maximum advancement of the facial skeleton and maintenance of a functional occlusion and acceptable aesthetics are the goals of surgical-orthodontic correction.[26] The author reports his experience with integration of virtual surgical planning (VSP) and the treatment of OSA with MMA surgery. Although VSP has previously been reported for treating skeletal-dental abnormalities and dental implant surgery, a paucity of knowledge exists reporting the feasibility and resultant outcome measures when virtual surgical planning is used for planning maxillary and mandibular surgery for patients with OSA. A case series of 4 subjects with a mean RDI and AHI of 86.1 and 75.5 events per hour, respectively, and an LSAT of 73% underwent MMA either as a phased approach or as a single treatment. Postoperatively, the mean RDI and AHI improved to 4.53 and 2.70 events per hour, respectively (P<.008), with an LSAT of 87%. Significant improvement in the posterior airway space at the occlusal and mandibular planes were achieved, P<.05, and the tooth-to-lip measurement was preserved (P = .92). VSP is a feasible tool used for predicting surgical outcome measures in MMA surgery for patients with OSA.[34]

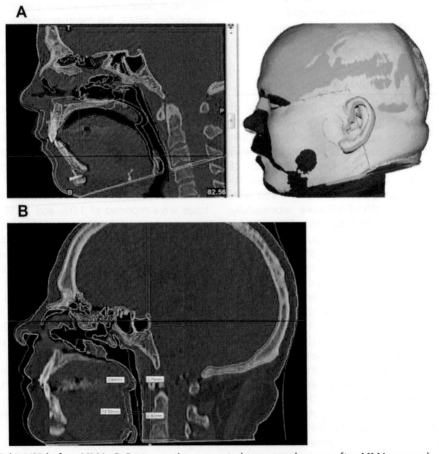

Fig. 6. VSP (A: VSP before MMA; B: Postoperative computed tomography scan after MMA surgery).

CASE STUDY

A 40-year-old man with severe OSA, notably an AHI of 70.9 events per hour, LSAT of 75%, RDI of 88.1, and ESS of 13 presented for surgical evaluation after PAP failure. His BMI was 29.3 kg/m². He underwent an uvulopalatal flap and geniotubercle advancement with a resultant improvement to AHI 13.3, LSAT 89% (<5 min), RDI 66.4, and ESS 12 with a BMI of 30.78. Due to his continued OSA and cognitive derangement, he underwent MMA surgery. VSP was performed to evaluate the patient and the patient underwent MMA based on the VSP.

His resultant PSG performed 17 months postoperative showed an AHI of 2.6 events per hour, LSAT 84% (<1 minute), and RDI of 3.7 with a BMI of 27.5 kg/m². The improvement in occlusal and mandibular airway measures were significant, 3.74 to 9.84 mm and 8.92 to 12.3 mm, respectively, P<.05. Tooth-to-lip measures were not significantly affected despite the achieved 8-mm advancement in the maxilla and mandible with 3-mm impaction, while the preoperative facial aesthetic profile was preserved (**Fig. 6**).

SUMMARY

A multilevel and phased approach based on the patient's level of obstruction has increased sleep surgery's overall success in reducing the severity of OSA.[1–3] This logical, stepwise approach identifies patients who demonstrate retropalatal and/or hypopharyngeal obstruction. GA, SG, hyoid myotomy and suspension, and MMA address retrolingual obstruction, and may be used alone or in combination with other upper airway surgeries, most commonly UPPP. The goal of surgery is to improve airflow around the base of tongue and reduce the number of obstructive events that occur during sleep. MMA has reported the highest success and cure rates of all procedures but must be tailored to the appropriate patient.

REFERENCES

1. Riley R, Guilleminault C, Powell N, et al. Mandibular osteotomy and hyoid bone advancement for obstructive sleep apnea: a case report. Sleep 1984;7(1):79–82.
2. Lewis MR, Ducic Y. Genioglossus muscle advancement with the genioglossus bone advancement technique for base of tongue obstruction. J Otolaryngol 2003;32(3):168–73.
3. Emara TA, Omara TA, Shouman WM. Modified genioglossus advancement and uvulopalatopharyngoplasty in patients with obstructive sleep apnea. Otolaryngol Head Neck Surg 2011;145(5):865–71.
4. Riley RW, Powell NB, Guilleminault C. Inferior sagittal osteotomy of the mandible with hyoid myotomy-suspension: a new procedure for obstructive sleep apnea. Otolaryngol Head Neck Surg 1986;94(5):589–93.
5. den Herder C, van Tinteren H, de Vries N. Sleep endoscopy versus Mallampati score in sleep apnea and scoring. Laryngoscope 2005;115:735–9.
6. Rodriguez-Bruno K, Goldberg AN, McCulloch CE, et al. Test-retest reliability of drug-induced sleep endoscopy. Otolaryngol Head Neck Surg 2009;140:646–51.
7. Barrera JE, Holbrook HS, Santos J, et al. Sleep MRI: novel technique to identify airway obstruction in obstructive sleep apnea. Otolaryngol Head Neck Surg 2009;140:423–5.
8. Barrera JE. Sleep magnetic resonance imaging: dynamic characteristics of the airway during sleep in obstructive sleep apnea. Laryngoscope 2011;121:1327–35.
9. Partinen M, Quera-Salva MA, Jamieson A, et al. Obstructive sleep apnea and cephalometric roentgenograms: the role of anatomic upper airway abnormalities in the definition of abnormal breathing during sleep. Chest 1988;93:1199–205.
10. Fujita S, Conway W, Zorick F, et al. Surgical correction of anatomic abnormalities in obstructive sleep apnea syndrome: uvulopalatopharyngoplasty. Otolaryngol Head Neck Surg 1981;89:923–34.
11. Riley RW, Powell NB, Guilleminault C. Maxillary, mandibular, and hyoid advancement for treatment of obstructive sleep apnea: a review of 40 patients. J Oral Maxillofac Surg 1990;48:20–6.
12. Riley RW, Powell NB, Guilleminault C. Inferior mandibular osteotomy and hyoid myotomy suspension for obstructive sleep apnea: a review of 55 patients. J Oral Maxillofac Surg 1989;47:159–64.
13. Riley RW, Powell NB, Guilleminault C. Obstructive sleep apnea and the hyoid: a revised surgical procedure. Otolaryngol Head Neck Surg 1994;111:717–21.
14. Waite PD, Wooten V, Lachner J, et al. Maxillomandibular advancement surgery in 23 patients with obstructive sleep apnea syndrome. J Oral Maxillofac Surg 1989;47:1256–61.
15. Riley RW, Powell NB, Guilleminault C. Obstructive sleep apnea syndrome: a review of 306 consecutively treated surgical patients. Otolaryngol Head Neck Surg 1993;108:117–25.
16. Hochban W, Conradt R, Brandenburg U, et al. Surgical maxillofacial treatment of obstructive sleep apnea. Plast Reconstr Surg 1997;99:619–26 [discussion: 627–8].
17. Prinsell JR. Maxillomandibular advancement surgery in a site-specific treatment approach for obstructive sleep apnea in 50 consecutive patients. Chest 1999;116:1519–29.

18. Lee NR, Givens CD Jr, Wilson J, et al. Staged surgical treatment of obstructive sleep apnea syndrome: a review of 35 patients. J Oral Maxillofac Surg 1999; 57:382–5.

19. Bettega G, Pepin JL, Veale D, et al. Obstructive sleep apnea syndrome fifty-one consecutive patients treated by maxillofacial surgery. Am J Respir Crit Care Med 2000;162:641–9.

20. Riley RW, Powell NB, Guilleminault C, et al. Obstructive sleep apnea syndrome following surgery for mandibular prognathism. J Oral Maxillofac Surg 1987;45:450–2.

21. Barrera JE, Riley RW, Powell NB. Facial skeletal surgery in the management of adult obstructive sleep apnea syndrome. Clin Plast Surg 2007;34: 565–73.

22. Andrews J, Barrera JE. Does tension matter? A study of tension in geniotubercle advancement surgery. Otolaryngol Head Neck Surg 2012;145(2 Suppl):P270.

23. Kezirian EJ, Goldberg AN. Hypopharyngeal surgery in obstructive sleep apnea: an evidence-based medicine review. Arch Otolaryngol Head Neck Surg 2006;132:206–13.

24. Rohrer J, Eller R, Santillan PG, et al. Geniotubercle advancement with a uvulopalatal flap and its effect on swallow function in obstructive sleep apnea. Laryngoscope 2015;125:758–61.

25. Hendler BH, Costello BJ, Silverstein K, et al. A protocol for uvulaopalatpharyngoplasty, mortised genioplasty, and maxillomandibular advancement in patients with obstructive sleep apnea: an analysis of 40 cases. J Oral Maxillofac Surg 2001;59:892–9 [discussion: 898–9].

26. Tiner BD, Waite PD. Surgical and nonsurgical management of obstructive sleep apnea. In: Miloro M, Ghali GE, Larsen PE, et al, editors. Peterson's principles of oral maxillofacial surgery. 2nd edition. BC Becker; 2004. Chapter 63. p. 1536–46.

27. Dattilo DJ, Aynechi M. Modification of the anterior mandibular osteotomy for genioglossus advancement with hyoid suspension for obstructive sleep apnea. J Oral Maxillofac Surg 2007;65(9):1876–9.

28. Handler E, Hamans E, Goldberg AN, et al. Tongue suspension: an evidence base review and comparison to hypopharyngeal surgery in OSA. Laryngoscope 2014;124:329–36.

29. Riley RW, Powell NB, Guilleminault C. Obstructive sleep apnea syndrome: a surgical protocol for dynamic upper airway reconstruction. J Oral Maxillofac Surg 1993;51:742–7 [discussion: 748–9].

30. Caples SM, Rowley JA, Prinsell JR, et al. Surgical modifications of the upper airway for obstructive sleep apnea in adults: a systematic review and meta-analysis. Sleep 2010;33(10):1396–407.

31. Holty JE, Guillenminault C. Maxillomandibular advancement for the treatment of obstructive sleep apnea: a systematic review and meta-analysis. Sleep Med Rev 2010;14(5):287–97.

32. Louis PJ, Waite PD, Austin RB. Long-term skeletal stability after rigid fixation of Le Fort I osteotomies with advancements. Int J Oral Maxillofac Surg 1993;22:82–6.

33. Nimkarn Y, Miles PG, Waite PD. Maxillomandibular advancement surgery in obstructive sleep apnea syndrome patients: long-term surgical stability. J Oral Maxillofac Surg 1995;53:1414–8 [discussion: 1418–9].

34. Barrera JE. Virtual surgical planning improves the predictability of surgical outcomes measures in obstructive sleep apnea surgery. Laryngoscope 2014;124:1259–66.

Controversies in Obstructive Sleep Apnea Surgery

Carolyn C. Dicus Brookes, DMD, MD[a],*,
Scott B. Boyd, DDS, PhD[b]

KEYWORDS

- Obstructive sleep apnea • Upper airway obstruction • Continuous positive airway pressure
- Polysomnography • Maxillomandibular advancement (MMA) • Surgical management/treatment

KEY POINTS

- Obstructive sleep apnea (OSA) is a common chronic disease characterized by repetitive pharyngeal collapse during sleep.
- Untreated OSA results in sleep fragmentation, which leads to excessive daytime somnolence. Untreated OSA is associated with decreased quality of life, increased risk of cardiovascular disease and all-cause mortality, and impaired cognitive function.
- Continuous positive airway pressure (CPAP) is first line therapy for OSA, but is not always tolerated. Alternative treatments are reviewed.
- Dynamic assessment of the airway in the OSA patient allows targeted intervention and plays a crucial role in surgical planning.
- Maxillomandibular advancement (MMA) is the most successful surgical intervention for OSA aside from tracheostomy; outcomes have been equated to those with CPAP.
- Multiple controversies and unresolved questions surrounding OSA remain and are explored in this article.

Obstructive sleep apnea (OSA) is a common chronic disease characterized by repetitive pharyngeal collapse during sleep. The estimated prevalence of OSA in middle-aged adults is between 20% and 25%,[1,2] and the overall prevalence of moderate to severe OSA is estimated to be 6.7% to 10.0%.[2,3]

Untreated OSA results in sleep fragmentation, which decreases time in deep sleep and leads to excessive daytime somnolence. Hypoxia and hypercarbia occur, and sympathetic activation increases.[4–6] Decreased vigilance, motor coordination, and executive functioning may result.[7] Depression[8] and decreased quality of life[9] may be seen. Untreated OSA has also been linked to hypertension,[1,10–12] arrhythmias,[10,12] congestive heart failure,[12] and increased risk of cardiovascular events,[13] as well as type 2 diabetes mellitus.[14,15] Stroke and all-cause mortality are associated with untreated OSA; risk seems to increase with OSA severity.[16] Because of the significant impact of untreated moderate to severe OSA, there is no question that treatment is indicated.

DIAGNOSIS

OSA is diagnosed based on polysomnography (PSG). This multimodal analysis reports several

This article was previously published in volume 29, issue 4 (November 2017) of *Oral and Maxillofacial Surgery Clinics of North America*.

The authors have no disclosures.

[a] Division of Oral and Maxillofacial Surgery, Froedtert & the Medical College of Wisconsin, CFAC 5th Floor, 9200 W Wisconsin Avenue, Milwaukee, WI 53226, USA; [b] Vanderbilt University School of Medicine, 1161 21st Avenue S, Nashville, TN 37232, USA

* Corresponding author.

E-mail address: cbrookes@mcw.edu

Sleep Med Clin 13 (2018) 559–569

https://doi.org/10.1016/j.jsmc.2018.07.005

metrics, among which are the apnea hypopnea index (AHI), respiratory disturbance index (RDI), nadir oxygen saturation, and percentage of time spent with oxygen saturation below specified thresholds. Severity of OSA is based on the AHI or RDI (mild OSA: 5–15 events per hour, moderate OSA: >15–30 events per hour, severe OSA: >30 events per hour), although other metrics must be considered during patient assessment. Per the American Association of Sleep Medicine, streamlined, more convenient and cost-effective home studies may be used in patients with a high pretest probability of moderate to severe OSA without certain comorbidities.[17] Additional components of the diagnostic evaluation are discussed later in this article.

NONOPERATIVE TREATMENT OF OBSTRUCTIVE SLEEP APNEA

Continuous positive airway pressure (CPAP) is the first-line treatment for OSA; it works by splinting the upper airway open to improve patency during sleep. When used appropriately and regularly, CPAP is highly effective for most patients. CPAP virtually eliminates OSA[18] and improves quality of life and sleepiness.[5,19,20] Unfortunately, nonadherence rates (with adherence defined as CPAP use for 4 or more hours nightly) of 46% to 83% have been reported.[21] Multiple mask designs and alternative positive airway pressure (PAP) delivery modes (eg auto-PAP) are available, and should be explored to help improve adherence. Intranasal steroids and nasal surgery may also improve PAP tolerance. The surgical provider should help encourage PAP use if possible. Nonetheless, treatment alternatives are necessary for patients who refuse or cannot tolerate CPAP.

Oral appliances (OAs) improve the upper airway by modifying the position of the tongue and associated upper airway structures. Custom, titratable, tooth-borne appliances designed to advance the mandible are the preferred OA.[22] OAs reduce AHI and improve nadir SpO2, although to a lesser degree than CPAP.[22] They improve sleepiness, control of hypertension, and quality of life.[22] Adherence to OAs appears to be similar to or slightly higher than adherence to CPAP.[23] OAs tend to work better for nonobese patients with skeletofacial deformities,[24] and patients must have reasonable protrusive range of motion to derive benefit from OAs. Monitoring for dental and skeletal changes is requisite.[22,25]

Additional nonoperative management strategies include positional aids if AHI is worse in the supine position,[5] sleep hygiene (including avoidance of alcohol, caffeine, and screen time before bed),[5]

and weight loss. A 10% weight loss has been linked to a 26% reduction in AHI[26]; however, OSA can recur even in the absence of weight gain, so follow-up is crucial.[27] Bariatric surgery may be used to help facilitate weight loss, and has also been linked to a decrease in AHI.[28]

Sleepiness that is unresponsive to OSA therapy may be managed by modafinil as long as other causes of daytime somnolence have been ruled out.[5]

SURGICAL TREATMENT OF OBSTRUCTIVE SLEEP APNEA

Many surgical approaches to adult OSA have been described. The more common are briefly reviewed.

Tracheostomy bypasses the upper airway and is thus nearly universally successful in managing OSA. However, the significant morbidity associated with tracheostomy limits its application in the OSA population.[29]

Bariatric surgery, as mentioned previously, is a surgical option in patients with morbid obesity.

Tonsillectomy with adenoidectomy is the first-line surgical therapy for children with OSA without craniofacial anomalies.

Nasal surgery may play a role in OSA management by improving nasal airflow. Particularly for those with moderate to severe sleep apnea, isolated nasal surgery is unlikely to lead to resolution of OSA. However, it may increase CPAP use in some patients.[30]

Multiple palatal procedures have been described; the most common is uvulopalatopharyngoplasty (UPPP), which involves removal of the tonsils, uvula, and posterior velum. Multiple variations of UPPP have been described. One meta-analysis reported a mean reduction in AHI of 33% to a mean postoperative AHI of 29.8[31]; however, UPPP does not reliably result in AHI normalization and is thus not recommended by the American Academy of Sleep Medicine (AASM) as a sole procedure for treating moderate to severe OSA.[32] A recent meta-analysis evaluated predictors for successful UPPP and found that only Friedman stage I (large tonsils and relatively normal palatal position) predicted surgical success; Friedman stage III and low hyoid position were negative predictors.[33]

Myriad tongue base procedures, robotic or conventional, have been described and may involve partial glossectomy or various ablative techniques to volumetrically reduce the tongue. Reported surgical success varies from 20% to 83%.[34]

Genioglossal advancement (GA) involves advancement of the genial tubercles, and may be accompanied by hyoid suspension. In conjunction with other therapies addressing palatal obstruction (or for those with isolated collapse at the retrolingual level) these interventions may be helpful. Multilevel surgery may be performed concomitantly or in a staged fashion. The AASM acknowledges multilevel surgery as an acceptable option for patients with multisite obstruction, but notes that the quality of evidence is low.[32] Reported surgical success rates for GA with or without hyoid suspension in conjunction with palatal surgery vary widely from 22% to 78%[34]; success rates seem to drop in the long term (65.2% vs 78.3% in one series).[35] Many procedures may be involved in multilevel surgical treatment of OSA, and less invasive combination procedures such as nasal surgery, palatal stiffening (eg, with implants) and radiofrequency ablation of the tongue have been reported on with a short-term success rate of 47.5%. The success rate in this series was higher for those with a body mass index (BMI) less than 30 kg/m^2.[36] A recent meta-analysis of radiofrequency ablation (RFA) for OSA found that most data were on management of mild-moderate OSA. Multilevel RFA showed an overall 41% reduction in RDI.[37]

Hypoglossal nerve stimulators are a relatively new addition to the array of surgical options for treatment of OSA, and were approved by the Food and Drug Administration for treatment of moderate to severe OSA in 2014. Postoperative titration is required. A multicenter trial reported surgical success in 74% at 3 years, although not all recipients used the device nightly[38]; another study reported 55% surgical success at 1 year postimplantation.[39] The device seems to improve symptoms and quality of life.[38,39] Hypoglossal nerve stimulation seems to be more successful when AHI is less than 50 in patients with a lower BMI and an anteroposterior pattern of palatal collapse.[40,41]

Maxillomandibular advancement (MMA) is the most successful surgical intervention for OSA aside from tracheostomy. MMA has been equated to CPAP in terms of outcomes. This procedure involves advancement of both jaws and addresses airway obstruction at multiple levels; airway collapsibility decreases due to advancement of its skeletal framework.[42] Its high success rate is likely because most patients with moderate-severe OSA exhibit multilevel obstruction.[43,44] Because of its high success rate and increased utilization, many of the controversies addressed in the remainder of this article focus on questions surrounding MMA.

Additional controversies with broader applications that are explored include evaluation of the airway and definition of successful treatment.

WHAT IMAGING/AIRWAY ASSESSMENT MODALITIES SHOULD BE USED ALONE OR IN COMBINATION FOR DIAGNOSIS, TREATMENT PLANNING, AND OUTCOMES ASSESSMENT?

Assessing the level of upper airway obstruction is a critical component of evaluation and surgical treatment planning for the patient with OSA, and has classically been done using awake nasopharyngoscopy. Additional imaging has been used to characterize the airway, to guide treatment planning, and to help assess outcomes.

WHAT IS THE ROLE OF LATERAL CEPHALOGRAMS?

Lateral cephalometric radiographs are readily obtained with low radiation, and may be used for preoperative planning before MMA. Attempts have been made to use them to predict levels of obstruction and anticipated treatment response to non-CPAP OSA therapies. However, lateral cephalograms have several important limitations when used for airway assessment.

A 2-dimensional image is inherently suboptimal for evaluation of a 3-dimensional structure, and lateral cephalograms for airway assessment are no exception. Clinically significant airway narrowing can be missed on a 2-dimensional view, which only demonstrates narrowing in the sagittal plane. Interestingly, lateral pharyngeal wall collapse has been linked to more severe sleep apnea than retropalatal and retrolingual collapse as assessed with dynamic MRI, and this change would not be noted on a lateral cephalogram.[45,46]

Airway measurements change throughout the respiratory cycle, so any measurements should be taken at a standardized point in the cycle. Even with every effort made to expose an image at a consistent point, though, different films could easily be taken at slightly different phases in the cycle. This could skew results when comparing measurements. Differences in head position at the time of imaging can also influence measurements.[47,48] Many individuals with OSA assume a head-up posture; it is important to obtain radiographs in a neutral head position.

Additionally, because lateral cephalograms are typically taken with the patient upright and awake, they do not characterize the asleep (or even supine) airway. The concept of supine cephalograms has been explored, but they are technically more challenging to obtain, which negates one of the main advantages of this imaging modality. Further, supine cephalometry still may not represent sleeping anatomy: An awake patient likely stents the airway when supine, and this may be more pronounced in the patient with OSA.[49]

Overall literature on the utility of lateral cephalograms in predicting treatment response to OAs, UPPP, multilevel surgery, or MMA is conflicting, with some studies showing no predictive value of various parameters, whereas others have linked specific measurements to success rates after various interventions. A recent review describes these studies nicely.[50] The role of cephalometry may continue to evolve; currently lateral cephalometric radiographs serve as an adjunctive airway assessment tool but cannot supplant direct airway assessment with endoscopy.

WHAT DOES 3-DIMENSIONAL CONE-BEAM COMPUTED TOMOGRAPHY AIRWAY ASSESSMENT ADD?

Three-dimensional airway assessment using cone-beam computed tomography (CBCT) has been used, and the addition of the third dimension offers an advantage over traditional plain films. When a CBCT is obtained as part of treatment planning for MMA, any data gleaned from the CBCT is available at no additional cost or potential harm to the patient. Although CT also can be used (and has the advantage of better soft tissue imaging), the additional radiation is difficult to justify. MRI is another option, but is used less frequently. Visually striking airway depictions make this modality particularly appealing in publications and to patients.

Multiple 3-D studies describe volumetric airway changes after MMA. These include increases in airway volume, minimal cross-sectional area, and both anteroposterior and lateral dimensions. Decreased airway length also has been shown,[51–54] as has anterosuperior movement of the hyoid.[55] Computational fluid dynamics can be used to assess theoretical airway flow and resistance, and this has been proposed as a method to predict surgical outcomes.[56–58] Increased airway volume after MMA has been linked to decrease in RDI and AHI,[51,55] although the magnitude of movement and changes in AHI are unlikely to fully correlate even with additional data because the dynamic nature of the airway is simply not accounted for when using this modality.

Despite increased data available on 3-D airway morphology before and after MMA and with use of OAs, there are limitations. As with lateral cephalometry, studies have reported data obtained in both the upright and supine positions. Measurements are similarly based on static images of the dynamic airway in awake patients, and respiratory phase and patient position may influence them.

Different anatomic boundaries may be used to define the airway; the impact of this is likely minimal, but still poses a challenge when comparing studies. The optimal interval from surgery to reassessment has not been defined, and the impact of time on results remains to be characterized. Perhaps most importantly, little is known about which parameters predict success with certain treatment modalities.

The primary roles of both lateral cephalograms and CBCTs remain characterization of baseline skeletal morphology and of postoperative skeletal changes. Three-dimensional airway analysis is likely to continue to be used primarily because it can be obtained from imaging taken for preoperative planning. It may contribute to our understanding of the airway in OSA and of the gross airway changes that result from various treatments, but it remains limited by its static nature, the challenges associated with precisely timing the image with respiratory cycle, and its exposure during the awake state.

WHAT ROLE DOES DYNAMIC UPPER AIRWAY IMAGING PLAY?

Dynamically assessing the level of upper airway obstruction in the patients with OSA allows targeted intervention and plays a crucial role in selecting a surgical procedure by allowing a description of the site, degree, and pattern of obstruction. It is also critical to rule out pathologic sources of obstruction, such as an obstructive tumor.

Awake nasopharyngoscopy with the Müller maneuver, or inspiration against closed nasal and oral airways, is used to assess level and degree of airway obstruction. Obstruction is scored by the observer but can be recorded for later review. Obstruction of more than 75% is typically considered severe and suggests the need for surgical correction at that site. The most significant limitation to this technique is that it is performed while the patient is awake.

Dynamic sleep MRI[45,59] and drug-induced sleep CT[44] have been used to characterize the airway in OSA. Advantages include the dynamic nature, the ability to evaluate the airway in a multiplane fashion, and the fact that these are obtained in the sleeping state or a simulated sleep state. One study explored airway differences between BMI-matched subjects with mild and severe OSA using sleep MRI; all subjects had retropalatal collapse, and all subjects with severe OSA had lateral pharyngeal wall collapse (vs <7% of those with mild OSA).[59] Lateral pharyngeal wall collapse as assessed by drug-induced sleep endoscopy has previously been correlated with hypoxemia in OSA.[60] This is one example of the type of information that may be derived from studies using these modalities. Although currently used in the research setting, these approaches may help further our understanding of levels of obstruction and impact of various treatments.

Drug-induced sleep endoscopy (DISE) has been introduced as an alternative to conventional endoscopy with the goal of more accurately representing patterns of collapse during the sleeping state. The introduction of DISE brings us closer to understanding the dynamic airway during sleep, but still has some shortcomings. The optimal anesthetic agent for DISE that most closely emulates the sleeping state has not been established,[61] and the results of DISE seem to vary based on agent used; for instance, propofol seems to lead to more airway obstruction and oxygen desaturations than does dexmedetomidine.[62] It seems that awake endoscopy and DISE detect retropalatal collapse equally well, but DISE may identify retrolingual collapse more often.[63] A systematic review reported that performing DISE after awake endoscopy changed the surgical plan in slightly more than 50% of cases, typically due to detection of additional hypopharyngeal or laryngeal obstruction. It is unclear, though, whether DISE improves surgical outcomes, and there is concern that DISE may lead to unnecessary surgical interventions.[61] More and more data are emerging about patterns of collapse on DISE that predict success with various surgical interventions and on DISE findings in treatment failures.

Accomplishing 3-D airway assessment while accurately reproducing the sleeping state has the potential to impact sleep apnea surgery significantly.

WHAT MEDICAL CONDITIONS PRECLUDE TREATMENT WITH MAXILLOMANDIBULAR ADVANCEMENT?

No definitive guidelines outline medical conditions that preclude MMA. As with any surgical procedure, the perioperative risk to the patient must be weighed against potential benefits, including risk reduction for sequelae of untreated OSA and improvement in quality of life. When in doubt, collaboration with the patient's medical team is paramount to guide decision making and, for the MMA candidate, to medically optimize the patient preoperatively.

First a decision must be made about whether the patient has sufficient reserve to tolerate a major procedure. Second, consideration must be given to medical comorbidities that could impact MMA in particular. For instance, severe osteoporosis could impact stability. Conditions with compromised wound healing, such as chronic immunosuppression or poorly controlled diabetes should be taken into account. Diabetes-associated microvascular and macrovascular disease could compromise blood supply, leading to loss of teeth, gingiva, or bone. Significant peripheral vascular disease, vasoactive drug use (eg, cocaine), or ongoing tobacco use can cause similar issues. Delay procedures could be considered in select cases to mitigate this risk. Conditions or medications that increase bleeding risk also merit consideration and, if surgery is pursued, require involvement of the appropriate specialists to guide management.

Uncontrolled hypertension should be optimized preoperatively. Baseline hypertension limits the safety of deliberate intraoperative hypotension, and can thus contribute to increased blood loss. This should be discussed with the patient and the anesthesia care team before surgery.

Uncontrolled or severe psychiatric disease may impact the patient's ability to adhere to postoperative guidelines and to integrate a new facial appearance. Preoperative discussion with the managing psychiatrist is crucial to ensure that management of psychiatric conditions is optimized and social support systems are in place. Careful consideration must be given to the use of steroids in this population.

There is no universally accepted age cutoff for candidacy for MMA, and general physical condition is more important than chronologic age. Age-related changes in sleep architecture should be incorporated into PSG interpretation. An additional consideration is that an older patient will likely enjoy the benefits of treatment for a shorter period, which may impact the risk-to-benefit ratio.

For some patients, alternative treatments must be explored to minimize surgical risk.

SHOULD MAXILLOMANDIBULAR ADVANCEMENT CANDIDATES BE OFFERED OTHER SURGICAL OPTIONS FIRST?

Initially a staged approach was recommended for surgical management of OSA. Phase I procedures included UPPP with or without adjunctive procedures, such as GA with or without hyoid myotomy, and phase II surgery involved MMA.[64] In theory this approach minimized morbidity while maximizing opportunity for successful outcomes. However, a recent comparative study confirmed that MMA alone is more effective than UPPP alone and reported that a traditional staged approach is no more effective than MMA alone.[65] Though UPPP is less morbid, its unpredictable success rate for those with moderate to severe OSA may make MMA as a primary treatment quite reasonable provided a patient can tolerate the larger procedure. Potential benefits of this approach over staged surgery for those who fail the latter include decreased total treatment time and earlier effective management of disease, a more favorable cost-to-benefit ratio, and reduced anesthetic and surgical risks.

Severe lateral pharyngeal collapse and laryngeal collapse on DISE have been linked to treatment failures in patients who received targeted interventions with multilevel surgery (most often palatopharyngoplasty and a base of tongue procedure); this cohort did not include patients who underwent MMA.[63] MMA, in contrast, has been shown to improve lateral pharyngeal wall collapsibility on DISE, and this change was correlated with surgical success.[46] Particularly for those with lateral pharyngeal collapse, strong consideration should be given to MMA as first-line therapy.

WHAT ARE THE INDICATIONS FOR ORTHODONTICS BEFORE MAXILLOMANDIBULAR ADVANCEMENT?

An absolute indication for preoperative orthodontics is patient desire to address a preexisting malocclusion in the absence of severe disease necessitating more urgent therapy. When a malocclusion is present that is not bothersome to the patient or when orthodontic therapy is not financially feasible, a discussion of potential benefits of definitive treatment of the malocclusion must take place. For instance, if a patient has a class II malocclusion or maxillary transverse hypoplasia, the patient should understand that orthodontic decompensation will allow further advancement of the mandible or widening of the maxilla, both of which may improve results. With baseline poor intercuspation, orthodontic treatment to improve dental relationships may enhance stability. However, it must be borne in mind that the goal of MMA is to treat a serious medical condition and to drop the associated risks; because of this, MMA without orthodontics may be pursued even if this yields a less optimal occlusal result.

The delay in MMA caused by orthodontic decompensation also must be considered, and patients should be strongly encouraged to adhere to nonsurgical treatment modalities and to strive for weight loss (if indicated) while awaiting skeletal sleep surgery. In some cases, early surgery (either before orthodontics entirely or before complete decompensation) may be performed, although this involves some guesswork on the final optimal jaw position.

When correction of a significant transverse deficiency is planned, surgically assisted rapid maxillary expansion (and/or surgical mandibular expansion) should be considered. A recent systematic review reported that maxillary expansion with or without mandibular expansion decreases AHI and improves nadir oxygen saturation.[66] The location of the transverse deficiency and stability will factor into selection of a surgical maxillary expansion versus a multipiece osteotomy.

IS THERE A ROLE FOR PREOPERATIVE SPEECH/SWALLOW ASSESSMENT BEFORE MAXILLOMANDIBULAR ADVANCEMENT?

No guidelines exist regarding preoperative speech assessment before MMA. Although regurgitation and hypernasal speech appear to be rare after MMA, improved ability to predict which patients might develop postoperative velopharyngeal insufficiency or swallowing dysfunction would be quite valuable. One systematic review noted that velopharyngeal insufficiency was reported only in patients who had undergone UPPP before MMA.[67] Patients with a history of palatal surgery should be counseled about the risk of velopharyngeal dysfunction. Consideration also could be given to preoperative speech/swallow assessment for those at high risk of postoperative dysfunction, such as individuals who have undergone previous palatal surgery.

WHAT IS THE IDEAL MAGNITUDE OF ADVANCEMENT IN MAXILLOMANDIBULAR ADVANCEMENT?

Scant data are available about the magnitude of advancement in MMA required to maximally benefit the patient with OSA. One frequently cited study suggests that mandibular advancement should be at least 10 mm.[68] However, a subsequent systematic review reported no association between degree of mandibular advancement and surgical success; data were analyzed at the study level and the patient level.[67] Study-level as well as univariate and multivariate patient-level analyses showed a higher surgical success rate with larger maxillary advancement (mean 9.9 vs 8.4 mm). The odds ratio for surgical success was 1.97 per 1 mm maxillary advancement based on multivariate analysis.[67] A recent small cohort study (n = 43 subjects) underwent smaller advancements (mean 5.2 mm in maxilla and 8.3 mm in mandible) with reported surgical success rate of 100% and surgical cure rate of 50% in the subset of patients with AHI data (n = 12).[69] These data suggest that the amount of advancement required to achieve surgical success remains poorly understood. Dynamic airway assessment may help improve our understanding of the optimal magnitude of advancement, and will ideally allow us to tailor this to each patient's needs.

WHAT ROLE DO ESTHETICS PLAY IN TREATMENT PLANNING FOR MAXILLOMANDIBULAR ADVANCEMENT? WHAT ARE SOME ALTERNATIVES TO CONVENTIONAL MAXILLOMANDIBULAR ADVANCEMENT?

Given the lack of literature supporting a specific magnitude of advancement, it seems prudent to factor in patient esthetics when planning the degree of advancement. This is particularly true in situations in which the patient is likely to develop an abnormal appearance after 1 cm of advancement and has less severe disease. Modifications to a straightforward maxillomandibular advancement also have been described and these or other variations can be applied to individual patients. Direct comparisons of outcomes with these different techniques are lacking.

Counterclockwise rotation of the maxillomandibular complex has been touted as a method to maximize mandibular advancement while minimizing the cosmetic impact of the surgery in the nasomaxillary region,[70] and may be appropriate for select patients. A recent meta-analysis demonstrated that both traditional and counterclockwise rotation result in a significant AHI reduction, but reported that there are insufficient data to determine superiority of either operation.[71]

A recently published alternative aimed at improving esthetic outcomes in the Asian face describes bimaxillary osteotomies coupled with anterior segmental maxillary setback; the result is advancement of the posterior maxilla with minimal effect on incisor position.[72]

Addition of a genioplasty can be esthetically beneficial, and should be offered if indicated. The potential airway benefits of genial tubercle advancement are discussed in the next section.

In the absence of strong literature support for one technique over another, careful discussion of the patient's goals and a detailed esthetic assessment should factor into decisions about the magnitude and direction of maxillomandibular movement as well as any additional modifications.

IS CONCOMITANT GENIAL TUBERCLE ADVANCEMENT OR NASAL SURGERY INDICATED DURING MAXILLOMANDIBULAR ADVANCEMENT?

In theory, genial tubercle advancement (either independently or as part of a genioplasty) may yield greater overall airway improvement. At present, though, there are few data to support the benefit of a genioplasty or genial tubercle advancement along with MMA on sleep parameters; this may be due to limited case numbers or a relatively small contribution of the genioplasty to AHI reduction. One review included 72 subjects who had undergone MMA with genioplasty as clinically indicated; there was no difference in AHI reduction or improvement in nadir oxygen saturation between those who had a genioplasty and those who did not.[65] A recent meta-analysis also showed that genial tubercle advancement in addition to MMA did not impact PSG outcomes.[73]

Concomitant nasal surgery may be considered to improve nasal airflow during MMA in select patients, although case selection is currently guided only by clinical judgment.

IS BONE GRAFTING DURING MAXILLOMANDIBULAR ADVANCEMENT BENEFICIAL?

Although some surgeons routinely graft during MMA, many do not. Good stability has been demonstrated with and without bone grafting.[68,74,75] If there are large lateral wall defects, autogenous or allogeneic grafts may be helpful. Grafting also may be helpful when treating the patient with an edentulous maxilla. Stepped osteotomies are advocated by some to ensure plates at the zygomaticomaxillary buttress are in thick bone while protecting the nasolacrimal apparatus medially.

HOW DO WE DEFINE TREATMENT SUCCESS?

Surgical success is classically defined as a 50% or greater reduction in AHI to less than 20 events per hour.[76] Surgical cure is defined as a reduction in AHI to less than 5 events per hour. Nadir oxygen saturation and percentage of time spent at a saturation below a threshold are among other metrics that merit consideration when evaluating polysomnographic changes. No consensus exists regarding optimal timing of the postsurgical PSG, although they are often obtained 3 to 6 months postoperatively to allow full surgical recovery and normalization of sleep patterns. Because OSA is a chronic, life-long disease, a long-term, durable treatment response is critical, and more information is needed about long-term outcomes.

The recently introduced effective AHI considers the time during which therapy is not used.[77] This is important when comparing interventions. For instance, MMA and CPAP result in similar AHI reductions.[78] However, CPAP and hypoglossal nerve stimulators may not be used for the entire sleep period, whereas MMA yields reduction in AHI during every hour of sleep. Taking this into account is crucial for outcome comparison.

Resolution of sleepiness, improvement in quality of life, and positive changes in cardiovascular health are also critical outcomes, and their incorporation into sleep medicine practices has been recommended by the AASM.[79] Sleepiness is most often assessed subjectively with the Epworth Sleepiness Scale.[5,80,81] Multiple quality-of-life questionnaires are also available; the Functional Outcomes of Sleep Questionnaire is an easily self-administered 30-question disease-specific quality-of-life assessment. It assesses several domains, including activity level, vigilance, intimacy/sexual relations, general productivity, and social outcomes.[82] Blood pressure and BMI are also important to follow, and are easily obtained.

WHAT ARE THE PREDICTORS OF SUCCESS OR FAILURE OF MAXILLOMANDIBULAR ADVANCEMENT IN TREATMENT OF OBSTRUCTIVE SLEEP APNEA?

One systematic review and meta-analysis of post-MMA outcomes concluded that, in addition to a larger maxillary advancement, a lower preoperative BMI was linked to an increased likelihood of surgical success.[67] Another meta-analysis of 45 studies including more than 500 subjects found that younger age and less severe preoperative OSA (as indicated by lower AHI and higher nadir SpO2) were associated with surgical cure. However, those with more severe preoperative OSA had a larger improvement in nadir SpO2 and a greater reduction in AHI than did those with a lower baseline AHI.[73] Although the surgical success and cure rates of MMA are quite high, we have much to learn about reasons for treatment failure.

SUMMARY

Although much is known about OSA, unanswered questions remain. Our understanding of the optimal airway evaluation in surgical candidates should continue to grow, as will our knowledge about predictors of successful treatment through various modalities. The inclusion of multiple outcome metrics in future case series in a more standardized fashion will also deepen our understanding of the impact of surgical treatment on individuals with significant OSA, particularly as reports on long term outcomes increase. Additionally, as reports emerge with larger sample sizes, we will develop a deeper appreciation for the impact of nuances in treatment planning on outcomes after MMA.

Multidisciplinary teams will lay the foundation for exploration of the unanswered questions in this field, and will facilitate delivery of the highest level of care to the CPAP-intolerant OSA population.

REFERENCES

1. Duran J, Esnaola S, Rubio R, et al. Obstructive sleep apnea-hypopnea and related clinical features in a population-based sample of subjects aged 30 to 70 yr. Am J Respir Crit Care Med 2001;163:685.
2. Peppard PE, Young T, Barnet JH, et al. Increased prevalence of sleep-disordered breathing in adults. Am J Epidemiol 2013;177:1006.
3. Young T, Peppard PE, Gottlieb DJ. Epidemiology of obstructive sleep apnea: a population health perspective. Am J Respir Crit Care Med 2002;165:1217.
4. Eckert DJ, Malhotra A. Pathophysiology of adult obstructive sleep apnea. Proc Am Thorac Soc 2008;5:144.
5. Epstein LJ, Kristo D, Strollo PJ Jr, et al. Clinical guideline for the evaluation, management and long-term care of obstructive sleep apnea in adults. J Clin Sleep Med 2009;5:263.
6. Somers VK, White DP, Amin R, et al. Sleep apnea and cardiovascular disease: an American Heart Association/American College of Cardiology Foundation Scientific Statement from the American Heart Association Council for High Blood Pressure Research Professional Education Committee, Council on Clinical Cardiology, Stroke Council, and Council On Cardiovascular Nursing. In collaboration with the National Heart, Lung, and Blood Institute National Center on Sleep Disorders Research (National Institutes of Health). Circulation 2008;118:1080.
7. Beebe DW, Groesz L, Wells C, et al. The neuropsychological effects of obstructive sleep apnea: a meta-analysis of norm-referenced and case-controlled data. Sleep 2003;26:298.
8. BaHammam AS, Kendzerska T, Gupta R, et al. Comorbid depression in obstructive sleep apnea: an under-recognized association. Sleep Breath 2016;20:447.
9. Reimer MA, Flemons WW. Quality of life in sleep disorders. Sleep Med Rev 2003;7:335.
10. Golbin JM, Somers VK, Caples SM. Obstructive sleep apnea, cardiovascular disease, and pulmonary hypertension. Proc Am Thorac Soc 2008;5:200.
11. Peppard PE, Young T, Palta M, et al. Prospective study of the association between sleep-disordered breathing and hypertension. N Engl J Med 2000;342:1378.
12. Phillips B. Sleep-disordered breathing and cardiovascular disease. Sleep Med Rev 2005;9:131.
13. Marin JM, Carrizo SJ, Vicente E, et al. Long-term cardiovascular outcomes in men with obstructive sleep apnoea-hypopnoea with or without treatment

with continuous positive airway pressure: an observational study. Lancet 2005;365:1046.

14. Vgontzas AN, Bixler EO, Chrousos GP. Sleep apnea is a manifestation of the metabolic syndrome. Sleep Med Rev 2005;9:211.

15. Wang X, Bi Y, Zhang Q, et al. Obstructive sleep apnoea and the risk of type 2 diabetes: a meta-analysis of prospective cohort studies. Respirology 2013;18:140.

16. Yaggi HK, Concato J, Kernan WN, et al. Obstructive sleep apnea as a risk factor for stroke and death. N Engl J Med 2005;353:2034–41.

17. Collop NA, Anderson WM, Boehlecke B, et al. Clinical guidelines for the use of unattended portable monitors in the diagnosis of obstructive sleep apnea in adult patients. Portable Monitoring Task Force of the American Academy of Sleep Medicine. J Clin Sleep Med 2007;3:737.

18. Giles TL, Lasserson TJ, Smith BH, et al. Continuous positive airways pressure for obstructive sleep apnoea in adults. Cochrane Database Syst Rev 2006;(3):CD001106.

19. Antic NA, Catcheside P, Buchan C, et al. The effect of CPAP in normalizing daytime sleepiness, quality of life, and neurocognitive function in patients with moderate to severe OSA. Sleep 2011;34:111.

20. Gordon P, Sanders MH. Sleep. 7: positive airway pressure therapy for obstructive sleep apnoea/hypopnoea syndrome. Thorax 2005;60:68.

21. Weaver TE, Grunstein RR. Adherence to continuous positive airway pressure therapy: the challenge to effective treatment. Proc Am Thorac Soc 2008;5:173.

22. Ramar K, Dort LC, Katz SG, et al. Clinical practice guideline for the treatment of obstructive sleep apnea and snoring with oral appliance therapy: an update for 2015. J Clin Sleep Med 2015;11:773.

23. Li W, Xiao L, Hu J. The comparison of CPAP and oral appliances in treatment of patients with OSA: a systematic review and meta-analysis. Respir Care 2013;58:1184.

24. Sutherland K, Vanderveken OM, Tsuda H, et al. Oral appliance treatment for obstructive sleep apnea: an update. J Clin Sleep Med 2014;10:215.

25. Goldberg R. Treatment of obstructive sleep apnea, other than with continuous positive airway pressure. Curr Opin Pulm Med 2000;6:496.

26. Peppard PE, Young T, Palta M, et al. Longitudinal study of moderate weight change and sleep-disordered breathing. JAMA 2000;284:3015.

27. Pillar G, Peled R, Lavie P. Recurrence of sleep apnea without concomitant weight increase 7.5 years after weight reduction surgery. Chest 1994;106:1702.

28. Ashrafian H, Toma T, Rowland SP, et al. Bariatric surgery or non-surgical weight loss for obstructive sleep apnoea? A systematic review and comparison of meta-analyses. Obes Surg 2015;25:1239.

29. Camacho M, Certal V, Brietzke SE, et al. Tracheostomy as treatment for adult obstructive sleep apnea: a systematic review and meta-analysis. Laryngoscope 2014;124:803.

30. Camacho M, Riaz M, Capasso R, et al. The effect of nasal surgery on continuous positive airway pressure device use and therapeutic treatment pressures: a systematic review and meta-analysis. Sleep 2015;38:279.

31. Caples SM, Rowley JA, Prinsell JR, et al. Surgical modifications of the upper airway for obstructive sleep apnea in adults: a systematic review and meta-analysis. Sleep 2010;33:1396.

32. Aurora RN, Casey KR, Kristo D, et al. Practice parameters for the surgical modifications of the upper airway for obstructive sleep apnea in adults. Sleep 2010;33:1408.

33. Choi JH, Cho SH, Kim SN, et al. Predicting outcomes after uvulopalatopharyngoplasty for adult obstructive sleep apnea: a meta-analysis. Otolaryngol Head Neck Surg 2016;155:904–13.

34. Kezirian EJ, Goldberg AN. Hypopharyngeal surgery in obstructive sleep apnea: an evidence-based medicine review. Arch Otolaryngol Head Neck Surg 2006;132:206.

35. Neruntarat C. Genioglossus advancement and hyoid myotomy: short-term and long-term results. J Laryngol Otol 2003;117:482.

36. Friedman M, Lin HC, Gurpinar B, et al. Minimally invasive single-stage multilevel treatment for obstructive sleep apnea/hypopnea syndrome. Laryngoscope 1859;117:2007.

37. Baba RY, Mohan A, Metta VV, et al. Temperature controlled radiofrequency ablation at different sites for treatment of obstructive sleep apnea syndrome: a systematic review and meta-analysis. Sleep Breath 2015;19:891.

38. Woodson BT, Soose RJ, Gillespie MB, et al. Three-year outcomes of cranial nerve stimulation for obstructive sleep apnea: the STAR trial. Otolaryngol Head Neck Surg 2016;154:181.

39. Kezirian EJ, Goding GS Jr, Malhotra A, et al. Hypoglossal nerve stimulation improves obstructive sleep apnea: 12-month outcomes. J Sleep Res 2014;23:77.

40. Van de Heyning PH, Badr MS, Baskin JZ, et al. Implanted upper airway stimulation device for obstructive sleep apnea. Laryngoscope 2012;122:1626.

41. Vanderveken OM, Maurer JT, Hohenhorst W, et al. Evaluation of drug-induced sleep endoscopy as a patient selection tool for implanted upper airway stimulation for obstructive sleep apnea. J Clin Sleep Med 2013;9:433.

42. Waite PD, Shettar SM. Maxillomandibular advancement surgery: a cure for sleep apnea syndrome. Oral Maxillofacial Surg Clin N Am 1995;7:327.

43. Kezirian EJ. Nonresponders to pharyngeal surgery for obstructive sleep apnea: insights

from drug-induced sleep endoscopy. Laryngoscope 2011;121:1320.

44. Li HY, Lo YL, Wang CJ, et al. Dynamic drug-induced sleep computed tomography in adults with obstructive sleep apnea. Sci Rep 2016;6:35849.

45. Liu SY, Huon LK, Lo MT, et al. Static craniofacial measurements and dynamic airway collapse patterns associated with severe obstructive sleep apnoea: a sleep MRI study. Clin Otolaryngol 2016;41:700.

46. Liu SY, Huon LK, Powell NB, et al. Lateral pharyngeal wall tension after maxillomandibular advancement for obstructive sleep apnea is a marker for surgical success: observations from drug-induced sleep endoscopy. J Oral Maxillofac Surg 2015;73:1575.

47. Muto T, Takeda S, Kanazawa M, et al. The effect of head posture on the pharyngeal airway space (PAS). Int J Oral Maxillofac Surg 2002;31:579.

48. Hellsing E. Changes in the pharyngeal airway in relation to extension of the head. Eur J Orthod 1989;11:359.

49. Martin SE, Marshall I, Douglas NJ. The effect of posture on airway caliber with the sleep-apnea/hypopnea syndrome. Am J Respir Crit Care Med 1995;152:721.

50. Denolf PL, Vanderveken OM, Marklund ME, et al. The status of cephalometry in the prediction of non-CPAP treatment outcome in obstructive sleep apnea patients. Sleep Med Rev 2016;27:56.

51. Abramson Z, Susarla SM, Lawler M, et al. Three-dimensional computed tomographic airway analysis of patients with obstructive sleep apnea treated by maxillomandibular advancement. J Oral Maxillofac Surg 2011;69:677.

52. Butterfield KJ, Marks PL, McLean L, et al. Linear and volumetric airway changes after maxillomandibular advancement for obstructive sleep apnea. J Oral Maxillofac Surg 2015;73:1133.

53. Fairburn SC, Waite PD, Vilos G, et al. Three-dimensional changes in upper airways of patients with obstructive sleep apnea following maxillomandibular advancement. J Oral Maxillofac Surg 2007;65:6.

54. Rosario HD, Oliveira GM, Freires IA, et al. Efficiency of bimaxillary advancement surgery in increasing the volume of the upper airways: a systematic review of observational studies and meta-analysis. Eur Arch Otorhinolaryngol 2016;274:587–8.

55. Hsieh YJ, Liao YF, Chen NH, et al. Changes in the calibre of the upper airway and the surrounding structures after maxillomandibular advancement for obstructive sleep apnoea. Br J Oral Maxillofac Surg 2014;52:445.

56. Sittitavornwong S, Waite PD, Shih AM, et al. Computational fluid dynamic analysis of the posterior airway space after maxillomandibular advancement for obstructive sleep apnea syndrome. J Oral Maxillofac Surg 2013;71:1397.

57. Yu CC, Hsiao HD, Lee LC, et al. Computational fluid dynamic study on obstructive sleep apnea syndrome treated with maxillomandibular advancement. J Craniofac Surg 2009;20:426.

58. Yu CC, Hsiao HD, Tseng TI, et al. Computational fluid dynamics study of the inspiratory upper airway and clinical severity of obstructive sleep apnea. J Craniofac Surg 2012;23:401.

59. Huon LK, Liu SY, Shih TT, et al. Dynamic upper airway collapse observed from sleep MRI: BMI-matched severe and mild OSA patients. Eur Arch Otorhinolaryngol 2016;273:4021.

60. Lan MC, Liu SY, Lan MY, et al. Lateral pharyngeal wall collapse associated with hypoxemia in obstructive sleep apnea. Laryngoscope 2015;125:2408.

61. Certal VF, Pratas R, Guimaraes L, et al. Awake examination versus DISE for surgical decision making in patients with OSA: A systematic review. Laryngoscope 2016;126:768.

62. Chang ET, Certal V, Song SA, et al. Dexmedetomidine versus propofol during drug-induced sleep endoscopy and sedation: a systematic review. Sleep Breath 2017. [Epub ahead of print].

63. Soares D, Folbe AJ, Yoo G, et al. Drug-induced sleep endoscopy vs awake Muller's maneuver in the diagnosis of severe upper airway obstruction. Otolaryngol Head Neck Surg 2013;148:151.

64. Riley RW, Powell NB, Guilleminault C. Obstructive sleep apnea syndrome: a surgical protocol for dynamic upper airway reconstruction. J Oral Maxillofac Surg 1993;51:742.

65. Boyd SB, Walters AS, Song Y, et al. Comparative effectiveness of maxillomandibular advancement and uvulopalatopharyngoplasty for the treatment of moderate to severe obstructive sleep apnea. J Oral Maxillofac Surg 2013;71:743.

66. Abdullatif J, Certal V, Zaghi S, et al. Maxillary expansion and maxillomandibular expansion for adult OSA: a systematic review and meta-analysis. J Craniomaxillofac Surg 2016;44:574.

67. Holty JE, Guilleminault C. Maxillomandibular advancement for the treatment of obstructive sleep apnea: a systematic review and meta-analysis. Sleep Med Rev 2010;14:287.

68. Riley RW, Powell NB, Li KK, et al. Surgery and obstructive sleep apnea: long-term clinical outcomes. Otolaryngol Head Neck Surg 2000;122:415.

69. Ubaldo ED, Greenlee GM, Moore J, et al. Cephalometric analysis and long-term outcomes of orthognathic surgical treatment for obstructive sleep apnoea. Int J Oral Maxillofac Surg 2015;44:752.

70. Brevi BC, Toma L, Pau M, et al. Counterclockwise rotation of the occlusal plane in the treatment of obstructive sleep apnea syndrome. J Oral Maxillofac Surg 2011;69:917.

71. Knudsen TB, Laulund AS, Ingerslev J, et al. Improved apnea-hypopnea index and lowest

oxygen saturation after maxillomandibular advancement with or without counterclockwise rotation in patients with obstructive sleep apnea: a meta-analysis. J Oral Maxillofac Surg 2015;73:719.

72. Liao YF, Chiu YT, Lin CH, et al. Modified maxillomandibular advancement for obstructive sleep apnoea: towards a better outcome for Asians. Int J Oral Maxillofac Surg 2015;44:189.

73. Zaghi S, Holty JE, Certal V, et al. Maxillomandibular advancement for treatment of obstructive sleep apnea: a meta-analysis. JAMA Otolaryngol Head Neck Surg 2016;142:58.

74. Lee SH, Kaban LB, Lahey ET. Skeletal stability of patients undergoing maxillomandibular advancement for treatment of obstructive sleep apnea. J Oral Maxillofac Surg 2015;73:694.

75. Louis PJ, Waite PD, Austin RB. Long-term skeletal stability after rigid fixation of Le Fort I osteotomies with advancements. Int J Oral Maxillofac Surg 1993;22:82.

76. Sher AE, Schechtman KB, Piccirillo JF. The efficacy of surgical modifications of the upper airway in adults with obstructive sleep apnea syndrome. Sleep 1996;19:156.

77. Boyd SB, Upender R, Walters AS, et al. Effective Apnea-Hypopnea Index ("Effective AHI"): a new measure of effectiveness for positive airway pressure therapy. Sleep 1961;39:2016.

78. Vicini C, Dallan I, Campanini A, et al. Surgery vs ventilation in adult severe obstructive sleep apnea syndrome. Am J Otolaryngol 2010;31:14.

79. Aurora RN, Collop NA, Jacobowitz O, et al. Quality measures for the care of adult patients with obstructive sleep apnea. J Clin Sleep Med 2015; 11:357.

80. Johns MW. A new method for measuring daytime sleepiness: the Epworth sleepiness scale. Sleep 1991;14:540.

81. Johns MW. Reliability and factor analysis of the Epworth Sleepiness Scale. Sleep 1992;15:376.

82. Weaver TE, Laizner AM, Evans LK, et al. An instrument to measure functional status outcomes for disorders of excessive sleepiness. Sleep 1997;20:835.

Transcranial Magnetic Stimulation
Potential Use in Obstructive Sleep Apnea and Sleep Bruxism

Herrero Babiloni A, DDS, MS*, Louis De Beaumont, PhD,
Gilles J. Lavigne, DMD, PhD, FRCD

KEYWORDS

- Transcranial magnetic stimulation • Sleep apnea syndromes • Sleep bruxism • Sleep medicine
- Sleep-disordered breathing

KEY POINTS

- Transcranial magnetic stimulation (TMS) is a neuromodulation technique with minimal side effects that has been used in obstructive sleep apnea (OSA) and sleep bruxism (SB).
- As an exploratory tool, TMS has been used to explore cortical excitability changes and other neuronal parameters, helping to understand pathophysiological mechanisms of both conditions.
- As a therapeutic tool and despite showing positive results, more research is needed before its validation as a treatment alternative.

INTRODUCTION

The objective of this article is to provide a basic understanding on transcranial magnetic stimulation (TMS) as well as to introduce to dental practitioners the use of TMS in dental sleep medicine, reviewing its mechanisms and applications to obstructive sleep apnea (OSA) and sleep bruxism (SB).

TRANSCRANIAL MAGNETIC STIMULATION
What Is Transcranial Magnetic Stimulation?

TMS is a noninvasive technique used to stimulate or modulate neural function.[1] Its mechanism of action is based on the principle of inductance, where electrical energy is obtained by passing a changing and powerful current through a coil positioned over the skull, producing a magnetic field that can excite neurons.[1] These neuronal effects can produce different physiologic and behavioral responses, depending on the targeted area of the brain and the type of stimulation.[2]

From a simplistic perspective, TMS can excite or inhibit neurons.[3] It is thought that the effects of TMS are mainly related to the cortex, but evidence suggest that TMS can also modulate activity from distant cortical and subcortical areas.[4–7] Nevertheless, the exact mechanism of action of TMS still remains debated.[8]

Types of Transcranial Magnetic Stimulation

Several different types of TMS paradigms have been developed over the past few decades, depending mostly on the number and frequency of pulses and the interpulse interval:

- Single-pulse TMS: consisting in single discharges separated by at least 4 seconds, to

Disclosure: Funding was provided by Canada Research Chair in Pain, sleep and trauma (G Lavigne) and Caroline Durand Foundation Research Chair in acute traumatology at University of Montreal (L De Beaumont).
Center for Advanced Research in Sleep Medicine, Hôpital du Sacré-Cœur de Montréal, 5400 Boulevard Gouin Ouest, Montréal, Québec H4J 1C5, Canada
* Corresponding author. CIUSSS Nord Ile Montréal, CEAMS E-1300, 5400 Boul Gouin O, Montréal, Québec H4J 1C5, Canada.
E-mail address: herre220@umn.edu

Sleep Med Clin 13 (2018) 571–582
https://doi.org/10.1016/j.jsmc.2018.07.002
1556-407X/18/© 2018 Elsevier Inc. All rights reserved.

avoid potential summation over time. This modality has been used mainly to evaluate corticospinal conduction disorders,[9] to map spatial distribution and somatotopic representation of muscles,[10] and to assess changes produced by physical activity[11] or light deprivation.[12]

- Double (paired)-pulse TMS: consists of a test stimulus that is preceded by a conditioning stimulus at an interstimulus interval of varying durations. This modality has been used to assess the conduction time between 2 brain regions, or interhemisphere inhibitory/excitatory processes.[13]
- Repetitive TMS (rTMS): consists of any combination of more than 2 pulses delivered with an interval of less than 2 seconds between the pulses. This modality is thought to have longer-lasting effects when compared with other paradigms.[1] It is thought to disturb neuronal communication[6] or increase cortical excitability,[14] making it a valuable modality from a therapeutic perspective.
- Theta burst TMS: is a type of rTMS that is shorter (20–190 seconds) in duration and that induces lasting effects on brain function.[15] It includes different paradigms and has shown promising results in certain conditions, such as major depression.[16]

Uses of Transcranial Magnetic Stimulation

Since it was first described in 1985 by Barker and colleagues,[17] TMS has been used for 3 main purposes[18]:

a. As an exploratory tool: to investigate the relationship between a cortical site and cognitive processes and behaviors; to understand the connectivity between brain regions during certain behaviors; to probe brain interactions during engagement in tasks; and to evaluate neuronal plasticity.

b. As a diagnostic tool: to estimate functional connectivity between or across brain hemispheres after brain lesions; to identify biomarkers.

c. As a therapeutic tool: to facilitate compensatory processes; such as neuronal plasticity and to remap and recover lost functions.

Clinical Applications of Transcranial Magnetic Stimulation

Different guidelines in the use of TMS for research and therapeutic purposes have been established.[1,19,20] It is thought that rTMS may present longer-lasting effects, thus becoming relevant for its possible therapeutic use, and specific rTMS have been developed,[21] presenting methodological recommendations for its use based on level of evidence (**Table 1**) derived from the value of the studies according to expert opinion (**Table 2**). These guidelines include several conditions, such as chronic pain disorders (neuropathic and non-neuropathic), movement disorders (Parkinson or Tourette syndrome, among others), stroke, multiple sclerosis, epilepsy, Alzheimer disease, and psychological disorders (depression, anxiety disorders) (**Table 3**). Although it is not the topic of this review, it is important to note the wide variety of clinical applications of TMS as well as its therapeutic potential.

Transcranial Magnetic Stimulation Safety

TMS is considered a safe, noninvasive brain stimulation technique with minimal side effects; the most common side effects being headache, and mild pain and discomfort in the skull.[19,20]

The main contraindication is the presence of ferromagnetic or metallic materials in contact with the coil. The rare occurrence of seizures has also been reported. Therefore, history of seizures,

Table 1
Level of evidence for transcranial magnetic stimulation application

Level of Evidence	Meaning	Requirements
A	Definitely effective or ineffective	At least 2 convincing Class I studies or one convincing Class I study and at least 2 consistent, convincing Class II studies
B	Probably effective or ineffective	At least 2 convincing Class II studies or one convincing Class II study and at least 2 consistent, convincing Class III studies
C	Possibly effective or ineffective	One convincing Class II study or at least 2 convincing Class III studies

No recommendation will be made in the absence of at least 2 convincing Class III studies providing similar results on the same type of clinical features with similar stimulation method.

Adapted from Lefaucheur JP, Andre-Obadia N, Antal A, et al. Evidence-based guidelines on the therapeutic use of repetitive transcranial magnetic stimulation (rTMS). Clin Neurophysiol 2014;125(11):2150–206; with permission.

Table 2
Value of evidence assessed and used by experts to classify repetitive transcranial magnetic stimulation studies

	Value of Evidence
Class I	Adequately data-supported, prospective, randomized, placebo-controlled clinical trial with masked outcome assessment in a representative population (n = 25 patients receiving active treatment). It should include a. Randomization concealment; b. Clearly defined primary outcomes; c. Clearly defined exclusion/inclusion criteria; d. Adequate accounting for dropouts and crossovers with numbers sufficiently low to have minimal potential for bias; e. Relevant baseline characteristics substantially equivalent among treatment groups or appropriate statistical adjustment for differences
Class II	Randomized, placebo-controlled trial performed with a smaller sample size (n <25) or that lacks at least 1 of the above-listed criteria a–e
Class III	Studies include all other controlled trials
Class IV	Studies are uncontrolled studies, case series, and case reports

Adapted from Lefaucheur JP, Andre-Obadia N, Antal A, et al. Evidence-based guidelines on the therapeutic use of repetitive transcranial magnetic stimulation (rTMS). Clin Neurophysiol 2014;125(11):2150–206; with permission.

brain injuries, anticonvulsant medications (such as carbamazepine, gabapentin, phenytoin), and medications that reduced epileptic threshold (narcotics, antidepressants, and antibiotics among others) should be taken into account before using TMS.[22] The risk in pregnancy, and in patients with severe or recent heart conditions or implanted cerebral electrodes is still uncertain.[22]

TRANSCRANIAL MAGNETIC STIMULATION IN OBSTRUCTIVE SLEEP APNEA
Obstructive Sleep Apnea

OSA is a sleep breathing disorder characterized by the narrowing of the upper airway that impairs normal ventilation during sleep (American Academy of Sleep Medicine guidelines). Clinically, it is defined by the presence of at least 5 obstructive respiratory events per hour of sleep (apneas, hypopneas, and respiratory effort–related arousals), accompanied by daytime sleepiness, loud snoring, witnessed breathing pauses, or awakenings due to gasping, or by the presence of 15 obstructive respiratory events without accompanying signs and symptoms.[23] The prevalence of OSA ranges between 7.0% and 49.7% in men and 3.0% to 23.4% in women.[24,25] Its diagnosis is made by clinical review of patient health, signs and symptoms, and by polysomnographic evaluation. Obesity seems to be the dominant risk factor,[26] and the consequences of nontreated OSA are higher risk of cardiovascular disease (hypertension, coronary artery disease, congestive heart failure, arrhythmias, and stroke), metabolic dysregulation, and diabetes.[27–32] The pathophysiological causes of OSA vary between individuals and include upper airway anatomy, the ability of the upper airway dilator muscles to respond to respiratory challenge during sleep, the propensity to wake from increased respiratory drive during sleep (arousal threshold), the stability of the respiratory control system (loop gain), and the potential for state-related changes in lung volume to influence these factors.[33,34]

Currently, the gold standard treatment for OSA is continuous positive airway pressure (CPAP), which has been shown to decrease mortality and morbidity of OSA.[35] However, adherence to treatment remains an issue for some patients. Other treatment options are behavioral strategies, such as weight loss, physical exercise, positional therapy, avoidance of alcohol and sedatives before sleep time; or oral appliances (OAs), which are indicated for mild and moderate apnea in patients unable to tolerate or who failed CPAP. OAs are considered a safe and tolerable therapy that can reduce morbidity and mortality in patients with OSA.[36] Adjunctive therapies, such as bariatric surgery, pharmacologic agents, and oxygen therapy also should be considered, as well as orthognathic surgery and uvulopalatopharyngoplasty for indicated cases. Other reported emerging therapies are upper airways stimulation, oropharyngeal exercises, nasal expiratory positive airway pressure, or oral pressure therapy.[37]

Applications of Transcranial Magnetic Stimulation in Obstructive Sleep Apnea

Studies that have used TMS in OSA can be differentiated into 2 main categories: those that used it as an exploratory tool to characterize the pathophysiology and mechanisms of OSA, and others that used it as a therapeutic tool to help improve OSA outcomes. Although the purpose of this

Table 3
Summary of clinical applications of repetitive transcranial magnetic stimulation with level of evidence A to C according to the guidelines published by Lefaucheur and colleagues, 2014[21]

Condition	Target Area	Level of Evidence	
		Low Frequency	High Frequency
Chronic neuropathic pain	Primary motor cortex, contralateral side of pain	Level B	Level A
Non-neuropathic pain	Primary motor cortex, contralateral side of pain		Level C
Parkinson disease	Premotor cortex, bilateral stimulation of hand and/or leg representation		Level C
Depression in Parkinson disease	Left dorsolateral prefrontal cortex		Level B
Stroke	Primary motor cortex	Contralesional postacute: Level C Contralesional chronic: Level B	Ipsilesional postacute: Level C Ipsilesional chronic: Level C
Hemispatial neglect	Posterior parietal cortex		Continuous theta burst stimulation contralesional: Level C
Epilepsy	Various cortical targets	Epileptic focus: Level C	
Tinnitus	Temporal or temporoparietal cortex contralateral	Single burst: Level C Repeated burst: Level C	
Depression	Dorsolateral prefrontal cortex	Right: Level B	Left: Level A
Posttraumatic stress disorder	Dorsolateral prefrontal cortex		Right: Level C
Auditory hallucinations	Temporoparietal cortex	Left: Level C	Left: Level B
Addiction/craving	Dorsolateral prefrontal cortex		Left: Level C

Applications with insufficient level of evidence are not listed in this table.
Data from Lefaucheur JP, Andre-Obadia N, Antal A, et al. Evidence-based guidelines on the therapeutic use of repetitive transcranial magnetic stimulation (rTMS). Clin Neurophysiol 2014;125(11):2150–206.

review is to give a general overview and not a detailed methodological description of the TMS protocols, more detailed information about TMS measurements and methodology can be found in **Box 1** and **Table 4**. One should note that there have been only a few studies on the topic and most had heterogeneous methodology, measurements, and outcome variables.

As an exploratory tool

TMS was used in patients with OSA and awake controls to characterize the responsiveness of the genioglossus and diaphragm, 2 muscles related to OSA, during respiratory and nonrespiratory faciliatory maneuvers.[38] The investigators found that when compared with controls, patients with OSA had different patterns of activity in the genioglossus and diaphragm (measured by motor evoked potentials [MEPs] and resting motor thresholds [RMTs]) after the different maneuvers, raising the possibility of a modification in the cortical control of these muscles during wakefulness, and highlighting the importance of studying them during sleep. Another study showed that patients with OSA presented increased motor connectivity (reduced MEP and central motor conduction time [CMCT]) of the genioglossus muscle during wakefulness at the end of expiration

---

Box 1
Definitions of transcranial magnetic stimulation (TMS) measurements provided in the literature

Motor evoked potentials (MEPs): Standard measure of motor response to TMS. It is an electrical potential difference detected using bipolar surface electromyography (EMG) over the target muscle.[76]

Resting motor threshold (RMT): Defined as the minimum stimulus intensity that produces a motor evoked response of at least 50 μV in 6 of 10 consecutive stimulations.[77]

Active motor threshold (AMT): Minimum stimulus intensity that produces a minimal motor evoked response of at least 50 μV in 6 of 10 consecutive stimulations when the muscle is contracted.[78]

Central motor conduction time (CMCT) or central conduction time (CCT): Is the time taken for neural impulses to travel through the central nervous system on their way to the target muscles. CMCT is calculated by subtracting the peripheral conduction time from the motor evoked potential latency elicited by motor cortical TMS.[79]

Cortical silent period (CSP): A pause in ongoing voluntary EMG activity produced by TMS. Although the first part of the SP is due in part to spinal cord refractoriness, the latter part is entirely due to cortical inhibition (seems to be mediated by GABA-B receptors).

Short afferent latency inhibition (SAI): Measures central cholinergic activity and the excitability and integrity of the sensorimotor system by delivering electrical stimuli to a peripheral nerve before a TMS pulse directed to the motor cortex.[80]

Short-interval intracortical inhibition (SICI) and long intracortical inhibition (LICI): Obtained with paired-pulse studies and reflects interneuron inhibitory influences in the cortex (thought to be GABA-A mediated).[81]

Intracortical facilitation (ICF): Also obtained with paired-pulse studies and reflects interneuron facilitatory influences in the cortex.[81]

Masseter inhibitory reflex (MIR): A bilateral, transitory interruption of the voluntary contraction of the jaw-closing muscles and is elicited by activation of the afferent fibers in the second and third branch of the trigeminal nerve, especially the mental nerve.[82]

---

when compared with age-matched and gender-matched controls.[39] The latter study also showed an association between increased motor connectivity and OSA severity. Although highly speculative and taking into account other electromyographic (EMG) studies,[40,41] the investigators proposed the potential existence of a central compensatory neural plasticity mechanism of the genioglossus muscle to the elevated upper airway pressure, which would increase muscular activity to keep the abnormal airway open during wakefulness.[39] In the same line, another TMS study compared the effect of hypercapnic stimulation on genioglossus and diaphragm muscles. However, the latter study did not find any alteration in corticomotor response of these muscles in patients with OSA.[42]

Other studies have also shown higher RMTs and longer cortical silent period (CSP) in untreated severe OSA,[43,44] as well as reduced MEPs and increased CSP during apnea episodes in patients with OSA,[45] suggesting an increase corticomotoneural depression and reduced cortical excitability. Some investigators have suggested that these cortical excitability alterations could be related to waking cerebral hypoperfusion and gray matter atrophy observed in patients with

OSA from previous studies.[39] These changes of brain structure and metabolism, which have been confirmed in subsequent studies, seem to be reversible with effective treatment.[46,47] Cortical hypoexcitability has also been observed in patients with OSA when compared with other sleep disorders, such as restless leg syndrome (RLS), indicating that the excitability of the cortex may be more affected in patients with OSA than in RLS.[48]

Other studies have attempted to increase cortical excitability using different TMS protocols. In a study using a high-frequency rTMS protocol (10 Hz, 1200 stimulations in total), which is known to increase cortical excitability of the stimulated brain region, patients with OSA showed reduced physiologic responses to rTMS (no modification of motor cortex [M1] cortical excitability and CSP duration) than controls.[44] As both reflect different physiologic mechanisms (increased MEPs size reflects the activation of N-methyl-D-aspartate receptors and lengthening of CSP is based on GABAergic tone), the investigators interpreted the latter study findings as an indication that patients with OSA had a widespread cortical alteration instead of a localized one. In another study, a continuous theta burst stimulation (cTBS)

Table 4
Methodological characteristics of studies using TMS in obstructive sleep apnea and sleep bruxism

Study	Condition	Status	Coil Location	Type	Main Measures	Main Results
Borel et al,[42] 2016	OSA	Awake	Genioglossus cortical representation	Single	Ventilation measures, MEPs (diaphragm, genioglossus)	No change in corticomotor response after hypercapnic stimulation
Civardi et al,[45] 2004	OSA	Awake, Sleep	FDI cortical representation	Single	RMT, MEPs, CSP (hand)	Reduced MEPs and increased CSP in apnea episodes in patients with OSA
Das et al,[44] 2013	OSA	Awake	FDI cortical representation	Single, rTMS (10 Hz)	RMT, MEPs, CSP (hand)	Reduced RMT, increased CSP, and lack of MEP/CSP rTMS response in OSA
Joo et al,[43] 2010	OSA	Awake	FDI cortical representation	Single, paired	RMT, MEPs, CSP, SICI, ICF (hand)	Increased RMT and CSP in OSA
Lanza et al,[48] 2015	OSA, RLS	Awake	FDI cortical representation	Single, paired	RMT, MEPs, CSP, SICI, ICF (hand)	RMT high in OSA, CSP short in RLS; OSA prolonged CMCT, MEP amplitude smaller in both
Melo-Silva et al,[52] 2013	OSA	Awake, Sleep	Submental cortical representation. (0–6 cm ant. 6–10 cm lat. to vertex)	Single	Respiratory variables, RMT, MEPs (submental)	Improvement airflow and inspiratory volume without arousing OSA
Melo-Silva et al,[53] 2013	OSA	Awake, Sleep	Submental cortical representation	Single (consecutive)	Respiratory variables, RMT, MEPs (submental)	Improvement airflow and inspiratory volume without arousing OSA
Nardone et al,[50] 2016	OSA	Awake	FDI cortical representation	Single, paired	Neuropsychological test scores, RMT, MEPs, CCT, SICI ICF, SAI (hand)	SAI reduced in OSA and strongly negatively correlated with neuropsychological test scores
Opie et al,[49] 2013	OSA	Awake	FDI cortical representation	Single, cTBS (3 stimuli at 50 Hz, repeated at 5 Hz for 40 s)	AMT, RMT, MEPs, SICI, LICI (hand)	Higher RMT and MEPs in OSA; No MEPs decrease after cTBS in OSA

Study	Condition	State	Target	Stimulation	Measures	Results
Rousseau et al,[54] 2016	OSA	Awake, Sleep	Submental cortical representation	Single, rTMS (1) 5 Hz-08s; (2) 25 Hz-02s; (3) 25 Hz-04s	Respiratory variables, RMT, MEPs (submental)	No airflow improvement with rTMS
Series et al,[38] 2009	OSA	Awake	Diaphragm: near vertex (2 cm anterior or 1 cm posterior to vertex); genioglossus: cortical representation	Single	Respiratory variables, MEPs during inspiration, respiration and tongue protraction (diaphragm, genioglossus)	OSA presents different genioglossus and diaphragm response patterns to facilitatory maneuvers, with some being related to frequency of sleep-related events
Versace et al,[51] 2017	OSA	Awake	FDI cortical representation	Single, paired	Olfactory test, RMT, SAI (hand)	SAI was reduced in OSA and negatively correlated with olfactory parameters
Wang et al,[39] 2010	OSA	Awake	Submental cortical representation	Single	MEPs, CCT (genioglossus)	MEPs latencies and CCT shorter in OSA, and CCT correlated with AHI at end of expiration
Gastaldo et al,[73] 2006	SB	Awake	M1 anterolateral orientation, parallel to central sulcus	Single, paired	AMT, MEPs, CSP, CCT, MIR (SP1 and SP2) in masseter	With paired stimuli, degree of CSP suppression was significantly lower
Huang et al,[74] 2014	SB	Awake	Masseter cortical representation (4–10 cm lateral to vertex and 0–4 cm frontal to biauricular line)	Single, paired	MEPs, MIR (SP1 and SP2) in masseter	With paired TMS recovery of SP2 was significantly lower in SB
Zhou et al,[75] 2016	SB	Awake	Masseter cortical representation	rTMS (1 Hz 20 min, 5 sessions)	Night EMG recordings, pain intensity (NRS), MEPs, AMT (masseter)	Decrease in pain and EMG activity during sleep

Abbreviations: AHI, apnea hypopnea index; AMT, active motor threshold; ant, anterior; CCT, central conduction time; CMCT, central motor conduction time; CSP, cortical silent period; cTBS, continuous theta burst stimulation; EMG, electromyography; FDI, first dorsal interosseous; lat, lateral; ICF, intracortical facilitation; LICI, long interval intracortical inhibition; MEP, motor evoked potentials; MIR, masseter inhibition reflex; NRS, numerical rating scale; OSA, obstructive sleep apnea; RLS, restless leg syndrome; RMT, resting motor threshold; rTMS, repetitive transcranial stimulation; SAI, short afferent inhibition; SB, sleep bruxism; SICI, short interval intracortical inhibition; SP, silent period; TMS, transcranial magnetic stimulation.

protocol, which normally reduces cortical excitability, was used to assess neuronal plasticity in patients with moderate to severe OSA.[49] In keeping with the previous high-frequency rTMS study, the findings showed an abnormal response to cTBS (lack of decrease in MEP) in patients with OSA, suggesting inefficient neural plasticity.

Another avenue for the use of TMS in OSA is the assessment of inhibitory cholinergic function in the cortex. This can be measured via protocols such as short afferent latency inhibition (SAI), which investigates sensorimotor integration regulated by the cholinergic system. It has been found that the SAI was significantly reduced in patients with OSA when compared with controls,[50] indicating a possible alteration of cholinergic function in patients with OSA. In addition, SAI measures were negatively correlated with higher scores in neuropsychological tests.[50] The investigators speculated that the latter finding may point toward a relationship between cholinergic and cognitive dysfunction. More recently, a study also reported a strong negative correlation between SAI measures and olfactory parameters in patients with OSA,[51] supporting the notion of a potential association between cholinergic neurotransmission and olfactory dysfunctions in patients with OSA.

As a treatment tool

It has been hypothesized that TMS could be used as a method to recruit upper airway dilator muscles (submental muscles) in patients with OSA to improve maximal inspiratory inflow during sleep while not waking the patient.[52] Five to 10 single, nonconsecutive TMS pulses were applied at the end of expiration and at the beginning of inspiration in 14 patients with moderate to severe OSA. During the night, CPAP was used at optimal-level pressure and at suboptimal-level pressure to induce flow limitation and evaluate TMS efficacy. Different levels of intensity were used, ranging from submental motor threshold to the lowest intensity consistently coupled with arousal (stimulation intensity increments varied between subjects). TMS stimulation was applied over the anterolateral area of the nondominant primary motor cortex (0–6 cm anterior and 6–10 cm lateral to the vertex) during non–rapid eye movement 2 sleep and during isolated (nonconsecutive) respiratory cycles. The investigators reported that TMS stimulation augmented maximal inspiratory flow and inspiratory volume of flow-limited respiratory cycles. They concluded that the TMS paradigm used allowed submental muscles to be recruited during sleep, increasing inspiratory patterns without arousing subjects with OSA. These results were also confirmed in a subsequent study

by the same group of investigators for consecutive respiratory cycles using the same stimulation protocol,[53] supporting the pertinence of TMS applied over the cortical representation of the submental muscles as a potential alternative treatment option for OSA.

The use of rTMS paradigms for recruitment of submental muscles in patients with OSA has also been explored by the same group to obtain more sustained results.[54] Three stimulation paradigms were applied at 1.2 of the sleep submental motor threshold intensity: (1) 5 Hz for 0.8 seconds; (2) 25 Hz for 0.2 seconds; and (3) 25 Hz for 0.4 seconds, over the same cortical area reported in their prior studies. Results showed no difference between baseline and post-rTMS measurements, which suggests that these rTMS protocols do not provide any airflow improvement of flow-limited breaths.

Summary

To summarize, TMS has provided new insights about the pathophysiology of OSA, pointing to irregularities in cortical excitability (mainly increased RMT and CSP), decreased neural plasticity (reduced physiologic responses to rTMS and cTBS stimulation protocols), and alterations in the cholinergic system (reduced SAI). Although a consecutive single-pulse TMS protocol has also emerged as a possible alternative treatment for some patients with OSA, early rTMS studies showed conflicting data. Obviously, more research is required to assess the efficacy of TMS as a management strategy for OSA.

TRANSCRANIAL MAGNETIC STIMULATION IN SLEEP BRUXISM
Sleep Bruxism

SB is considered an oral behavior in otherwise healthy persons[55] and also a sleep movement disorder, identified as a repetitive jaw muscle activity that is characterized by clenching or grinding of the teeth and/or by bracing or thrusting of the mandible.[56] Prevalence of SB has been estimated to be approximately 12.8%, with no predominance for sex and decreasing with age,[57] and despite being related to many physiological factors, such as sleep microarousals in young and otherwise healthy subjects,[58] its etiology remains unknown. The diagnosis of SB is based on clinical features, such as reports of tooth-grinding sounds, abnormal tooth wear, morning jaw muscle pain or fatigue, temporal headaches, or jaw locking on awakening.[23] However, this diagnostic approach may be not very accurate due to different sources of variability (eg, time to time, age).

Polysomnographic assessment is indicated when other sleep disorder is suspected. The consequences of SB are diverse and they are mainly dental, including dental attrition that can cause hypersensitivity, reduced vertical dimension (aesthetics), pulpitis, abfractions, and hypermobility, among others.[59] SB also has been associated with implant failure and periodontal disease progression, but systematic reviews did not seem to support these associations.[60,61] Muscle hypertrophy and transient morning headaches also have been considered consequences of SB, and despite recent evidence suggesting that resting jaw muscle tone can be among the risk factors of temporomandibular disorders (TMD),[62] the relationship between SB and TMD remains debated.[63–65]

Different treatment options have been used to manage this condition. For dentists, one of the best-known approaches is the use of OAs. Their exact mechanism of action is not well understood, but it appears that their use can be effective in managing the consequences of SB.[66] Another approach explored is the use of pharmacotherapy. Clonazepam and clonidine have more robust evidence for their oral administration, although risk of dependence and blood pressure lowering with consequent falls should be considered respectively.[67–70] Botulinum toxin injected intramuscularly is another medication that has gained in popularity in the recent years, even though studies report mixed results.[66] Other medications that were used with less success include propranolol, amitriptyline, pramipexole, bromocriptine, gabapentin, tryptophan, and levodopa.[66,71] Finally, other reported modalities are muscular electrical stimulation, biofeedback, cognitive behavioral therapy, or physical exercises, which also presented mixed results or still need to be adapted to a clinical use.[66,71,72]

Transcranial Magnetic Stimulation Applications in Sleep Bruxism

The use of TMS in SB is quite limited. To our knowledge, only 3 studies have used TMS in SB, 2 of them as an exploratory tool, and the other as a therapeutic tool (**Box 1** and **Table 4**).

Exploratory tool

Single and paired TMS stimuli were used to investigate motor cortex excitability during wake time in participants with SB in 2 studies during wakefulness.[73,74] MEPs in masseter muscles and the "recovery cycle" of the masseter inhibitory reflex (MIR), which was composed of early silent periods (SP1) and late silent periods (SP2), were analyzed and compared with controls in both studies. No difference in MEPs and SPs were found between groups with the single-pulse TMS. In contrast, with the double-pulse TMS, the recovery of SP2 was lower in patients with SB in the 2 studies, suggesting an increased cortical excitability.

Therapeutic tool

An open pilot trial with rTMS was conducted in 12 participants with SB, which was assessed by self-report (questionnaire) and by clinical examination.[75] The protocol consisted of 5 sessions (1 session on each day for 5 consecutive days) of 20 minutes of rTMS stimulation at 1 Hz, 80% intensity of active motor threshold (AMT) on both masseter representations of the somatosensory cortex during wakefulness and at rest. Masseter activity, measured through EMG intensity and bursts at night, and pain soreness due to muscle activity, measured by numerical rating scale (NRS), were assessed at baseline, during treatment, and at the 5-day follow-up. Study results showed a significant decrease in EMG recordings and NRS during treatment and at follow-up, suggesting that 5 sessions of rTMS at 1 Hz may be an effective therapeutic option to manage SB. However, the absence of a control group and the open design calls for caution in the interpretation of their results.

Summary

The use of TMS in SB seems to indicate alterations in cortical excitability. At this time, literature is very scarce to determine if TMS can be considered as a therapeutic tool to manage SB.

SUMMARY

For sleep disorders, such as OSA or SB, TMS has contributed (1) to understanding their pathophysiological mechanisms, exploring cortical excitability changes, and other neuronal parameters that may clarify the disorder; and (2) to guide future lines of research and/or management strategies. In both conditions, different modalities of TMS have shown positive results as a therapeutic option of management, but obviously this type of management tool needs further validation before its use can be accepted in clinical settings for OSA and SB.

REFERENCES

1. Wassermann EM. Risk and safety of repetitive transcranial magnetic stimulation: report and suggested guidelines from the International Workshop on the Safety of Repetitive Transcranial Magnetic Stimulation, June 5-7, 1996. Electroencephalogr Clin Neurophysiol 1998;108(1):1–16.

2. Horvath JC, Perez JM, Forrow L, et al. Transcranial magnetic stimulation: a historical evaluation and future prognosis of therapeutically relevant ethical concerns. J Med Ethics 2011;37(3):137–43.

3. Siebner HR, Rothwell J. Transcranial magnetic stimulation: new insights into representational cortical plasticity. Exp Brain Res 2003;148(1):1–16.

4. Paus T, Castro-Alamancos MA, Petrides M. Cortico-cortical connectivity of the human mid-dorsolateral frontal cortex and its modulation by repetitive transcranial magnetic stimulation. Eur J Neurosci 2001; 14(8):1405–11.

5. Chouinard PA, Van Der Werf YD, Leonard G, et al. Modulating neural networks with transcranial magnetic stimulation applied over the dorsal premotor and primary motor cortices. J Neurophysiol 2003; 90(2):1071–83.

6. Valero-Cabre A, Payne BR, Rushmore J, et al. Impact of repetitive transcranial magnetic stimulation of the parietal cortex on metabolic brain activity: a 14C-2DG tracing study in the cat. Exp Brain Res 2005;163(1):1–12.

7. Valero-Cabre A, Payne BR, Pascual-Leone A. Opposite impact on 14C-2-deoxyglucose brain metabolism following patterns of high and low frequency repetitive transcranial magnetic stimulation in the posterior parietal cortex. Exp Brain Res 2007;176(4):603–15.

8. Chervyakov AV, Chernyavsky AY, Sinitsyn DO, et al. Possible mechanisms underlying the therapeutic effects of transcranial magnetic stimulation. Front Hum Neurosci 2015;9:303.

9. Chen R, Cros D, Curra A, et al. The clinical diagnostic utility of transcranial magnetic stimulation: report of an IFCN committee. Clin Neurophysiol 2008;119(3):504–32.

10. Levy WJ, Amassian VE, Schmid UD, et al. Mapping of motor cortex gyral sites non-invasively by transcranial magnetic stimulation in normal subjects and patients. Electroencephalogr Clin Neurophysiol Suppl 1991;43:51–75.

11. Ziemann U, Muellbacher W, Hallett M, et al. Modulation of practice-dependent plasticity in human motor cortex. Brain 2001;124(Pt 6):1171–81.

12. Boroojerdi B, Bushara KO, Corwell B, et al. Enhanced excitability of the human visual cortex induced by short-term light deprivation. Cereb Cortex 2000;10(5):529–34.

13. Baumer T, Bock F, Koch G, et al. Magnetic stimulation of human premotor or motor cortex produces interhemispheric facilitation through distinct pathways. J Physiol 2006;572(Pt 3):857–68.

14. Fierro B, Brighina F, Vitello G, et al. Modulatory effects of low- and high-frequency repetitive transcranial magnetic stimulation on visual cortex of healthy subjects undergoing light deprivation. J Physiol 2005;565(Pt 2):659–65.

15. Huang YZ, Edwards MJ, Rounis E, et al. Theta burst stimulation of the human motor cortex. Neuron 2005; 45(2):201–6.

16. Berlim MT, McGirr A, Rodrigues Dos Santos N, et al. Efficacy of theta burst stimulation (TBS) for major depression: an exploratory meta-analysis of randomized and sham-controlled trials. J Psychiatr Res 2017;90:102–9.

17. Barker AT, Jalinous R, Freeston IL. Non-invasive magnetic stimulation of human motor cortex. Lancet 1985;1(8437):1106–7.

18. Valero-Cabre A, Amengual J, Stengel C, et al. Transcranial Magnetic Stimulation in basic and clinical neuroscience: a comprehensive review of fundamental principles and novel insights. Neurosci Biobehav Rev 2017;83:381–404.

19. Machii K, Cohen D, Ramos-Estebanez C, et al. Safety of rTMS to non-motor cortical areas in healthy participants and patients. Clin Neurophysiol 2006; 117(2):455–71.

20. Klein MM, Treister R, Raij T, et al. Transcranial magnetic stimulation of the brain: guidelines for pain treatment research. Pain 2015;156(9): 1601–14.

21. Lefaucheur JP, Andre-Obadia N, Antal A, et al. Evidence-based guidelines on the therapeutic use of repetitive transcranial magnetic stimulation (rTMS). Clin Neurophysiol 2014;125(11):2150–206.

22. Rossi S, Hallett M, Rossini PM, et al, Safety of TMS Consensus Group. Safety, ethical considerations, and application guidelines for the use of transcranial magnetic stimulation in clinical practice and research. Clin Neurophysiol 2009;120(12):2008–39.

23. American Academy of Sleep Medicine. International classification of Sleep Disorders. 3rd edition. Darien (IL): American Academy of Sleep Medicine; 2014.

24. Punjabi NM. The epidemiology of adult obstructive sleep apnea. Proc Am Thorac Soc 2008;5(2):136–43.

25. Heinzer R, Vat S, Marques-Vidal P, et al. Prevalence of sleep-disordered breathing in the general population: the HypnoLaus study. Lancet Respir Med 2015; 3(4):310–8.

26. Young T, Skatrud J, Peppard PE. Risk factors for obstructive sleep apnea in adults. JAMA 2004; 291(16):2013–6.

27. Marin JM, Carrizo SJ, Vicente E, et al. Long-term cardiovascular outcomes in men with obstructive sleep apnoea-hypopnoea with or without treatment with continuous positive airway pressure: an observational study. Lancet 2005;365(9464):1046–53.

28. Gami AS, Rader S, Svatikova A, et al. Familial premature coronary artery disease mortality and obstructive sleep apnea. Chest 2007;131(1): 118–21.

29. Budhiraja R, Budhiraja P, Quan SF. Sleep-disordered breathing and cardiovascular disorders. Respir Care 2010;55(10):1322–32 [discussion: 1330–2].

30. Lam JC, Mak JC, Ip MS. Obesity, obstructive sleep apnoea and metabolic syndrome. Respirology 2012;17(2):223–36.

31. Peppard PE, Young T, Palta M, et al. Prospective study of the association between sleep-disordered breathing and hypertension. N Engl J Med 2000; 342(19):1378–84.

32. Punjabi NM, Shahar E, Redline S, et al. Sleep-disordered breathing, glucose intolerance, and insulin resistance: the Sleep Heart Health Study. Am J Epidemiol 2004;160(6):521–30.

33. Eckert DJ, Malhotra A. Pathophysiology of adult obstructive sleep apnea. Proc Am Thorac Soc 2008;5(2):144–53.

34. Osman AM, Carter SG, Carberry JC, et al. Obstructive sleep apnea: current perspectives. Nat Sci Sleep 2018;10:21–34.

35. Epstein LJ, Kristo D, Strollo PJ Jr, et al. Clinical guideline for the evaluation, management and long-term care of obstructive sleep apnea in adults. J Clin Sleep Med 2009;5(3):263–76.

36. de Vries GE, Wijkstra PJ, Houwerzijl EJ, et al. Cardiovascular effects of oral appliance therapy in obstructive sleep apnea: a systematic review and meta-analysis. Sleep Med Rev 2017;40:55–68.

37. Lorenzi-Filho G, Almeida FR, Strollo PJ. Treating OSA: current and emerging therapies beyond CPAP. Respirology 2017;22(8):1500–7.

38. Series F, Wang W, Similowski T. Corticomotor control of the genioglossus in awake OSAS patients: a transcranial magnetic stimulation study. Respir Res 2009;10:74.

39. Wang W, Kang J, Kong D. The central motor conductivity of genioglossus in obstructive sleep apnoea. Respirology 2010;15(8):1209–14.

40. Mezzanotte WS, Tangel DJ, White DP. Waking genioglossal electromyogram in sleep apnea patients versus normal controls (a neuromuscular compensatory mechanism). J Clin Invest 1992;89(5):1571–9.

41. Fogel RB, Malhotra A, Pillar G, et al. Genioglossal activation in patients with obstructive sleep apnea versus control subjects. Mechanisms of muscle control. Am J Respir Crit Care Med 2001;164(11):2025–30.

42. Borel JC, Melo-Silva CA, Gakwaya S, et al. Diaphragm and genioglossus corticomotor excitability in patients with obstructive sleep apnea and control subjects. J Sleep Res 2016;25(1):23–30.

43. Joo EY, Kim HJ, Lim YH, et al. Altered cortical excitability in patients with untreated obstructive sleep apnea syndrome. Sleep Med 2010;11(9):857–61.

44. Das A, Anupa AV, Radhakrishnan A. Reduced plastic brain responses to repetitive transcranial magnetic stimulation in severe obstructive sleep apnea syndrome. Sleep Med 2013;14(7):636–40.

45. Civardi C, Naldi P, Cantello R. Cortico-motoneurone excitability in patients with obstructive sleep apnoea. J Sleep Res 2004;13(2):159–63.

46. Canessa N, Castronovo V, Cappa SF, et al. Obstructive sleep apnea: brain structural changes and neurocognitive function before and after treatment. Am J Respir Crit Care Med 2011;183(10): 1419–26.

47. Castronovo V, Scifo P, Castellano A, et al. White matter integrity in obstructive sleep apnea before and after treatment. Sleep 2014;37(9):1465–75.

48. Lanza G, Lanuzza B, Arico D, et al. Direct comparison of cortical excitability to transcranial magnetic stimulation in obstructive sleep apnea syndrome and restless legs syndrome. Sleep Med 2015; 16(1):138–42.

49. Opie GM, Catcheside PG, Usmani ZA, et al. Motor cortex plasticity induced by theta burst stimulation is impaired in patients with obstructive sleep apnoea. Eur J Neurosci 2013;37(11):1844–52.

50. Nardone R, Bergmann J, Brigo F, et al. Cortical afferent inhibition reflects cognitive impairment in obstructive sleep apnea syndrome: a TMS study. Sleep Med 2016;24:51–6.

51. Versace V, Langthaler PB, Sebastianelli L, et al. Cholinergic neurotransmission and olfactory function in obstructive sleep apnea syndrome: a TMS study. Sleep Med 2017;37:113–8.

52. Melo-Silva CA, Borel JC, Gakwaya S, et al. Acute upper airway muscle and inspiratory flow responses to transcranial magnetic stimulation during sleep in apnoeic patients. Exp Physiol 2013; 98(4):946–56.

53. Melo-Silva CA, Gakwaya S, Rousseau E, et al. Consecutive transcranial magnetic stimulation twitches reduce flow limitation during sleep in apnoeic patients. Exp Physiol 2013;98(9):1366–75.

54. Rousseau E, Melo-Silva CA, Gakwaya S, et al. Effects of repetitive transcranial magnetic stimulation of upper airway muscles during sleep in obstructive sleep apnea patients. J Appl Physiol (1985) 2016; 121(5):1217–25.

55. Raphael KG, Santiago V, Lobbezoo F. Is bruxism a disorder or a behaviour? Rethinking the international consensus on defining and grading of bruxism. J Oral Rehabil 2016;43(10):791–8.

56. Lobbezoo F, Ahlberg J, Raphael KG, et al. International consensus on the assessment of bruxism: Report of a work in progress. J Oral Rehabil 2018. [Epub ahead of print].

57. Manfredini D, Winocur E, Guarda-Nardini L, et al. Epidemiology of bruxism in adults: a systematic review of the literature. J Orofac Pain 2013;27(2): 99–110.

58. Kato T, Thie NM, Montplaisir JY, et al. Bruxism and orofacial movements during sleep. Dent Clin North Am 2001;45(4):657–84.

59. Yap AU, Chua AP. Sleep bruxism: current knowledge and contemporary management. J Conserv Dent 2016;19(5):383–9.

60. Manfredini D, Ahlberg J, Mura R, et al. Bruxism is unlikely to cause damage to the periodontium: findings from a systematic literature assessment. J Periodontol 2015;86(4):546–55.

61. Manfredini D, Poggio CE, Lobbezoo F. Is bruxism a risk factor for dental implants? A systematic review of the literature. Clin Implant Dent Relat Res 2014; 16(3):460–9.

62. Raphael KG, Janal MN, Sirois DA, et al. Masticatory muscle sleep background electromyographic activity is elevated in myofascial temporomandibular disorder patients. J Oral Rehabil 2013;40(12):883–91.

63. Fernandes G, Franco AL, Goncalves DA, et al. Temporomandibular disorders, sleep bruxism, and primary headaches are mutually associated. J Orofac pain 2013;27(1):14–20.

64. Jimenez-Silva A, Pena-Duran C, Tobar-Reyes J, et al. Sleep and awake bruxism in adults and its relationship with temporomandibular disorders: a systematic review from 2003 to 2014. Acta Odontol Scand 2017;75(1):36–58.

65. Raphael KG, Sirois DA, Janal MN, et al. Sleep bruxism and myofascial temporomandibular disorders: a laboratory-based polysomnographic investigation. J Am Dental Assoc 2012;143(11):1223–31.

66. Manfredini D, Ahlberg J, Winocur E, et al. Management of sleep bruxism in adults: a qualitative systematic literature review. J Oral Rehabil 2015; 42(11):862–74.

67. Saletu A, Parapatics S, Anderer P, et al. Controlled clinical, polysomnographic and psychometric studies on differences between sleep bruxers and controls and acute effects of clonazepam as compared with placebo. Eur Arch Psychiatry Clin Neurosci 2010;260(2):163–74.

68. Carra MC, Macaluso GM, Rompre PH, et al. Clonidine has a paradoxical effect on cyclic arousal and sleep bruxism during NREM sleep. Sleep 2010; 33(12):1711–6.

69. Huynh N, Lavigne GJ, Lanfranchi PA, et al. The effect of 2 sympatholytic medications—propranolol and clonidine—on sleep bruxism: experimental randomized controlled studies. Sleep 2006;29(3): 307–16.

70. Sakai T, Kato T, Yoshizawa S, et al. Effect of clonazepam and clonidine on primary sleep bruxism: a double-blind, crossover, placebo-controlled trial. J Sleep Res 2017;26(1):73–83.

71. Lobbezoo F, van der Zaag J, van Selms MK, et al. Principles for the management of bruxism. J Oral Rehabil 2008;35(7):509–23.

72. Jadidi F, Castrillon EE, Nielsen P, et al. Effect of contingent electrical stimulation on jaw muscle activity during sleep: a pilot study with a randomized controlled trial design. Acta Odontol Scand 2013; 71(5):1050–62.

73. Gastaldo E, Quatrale R, Graziani A, et al. The excitability of the trigeminal motor system in sleep bruxism: a transcranial magnetic stimulation and brainstem reflex study. J Orofac pain 2006;20(2): 145–55.

74. Huang H, Song YH, Wang JJ, et al. Excitability of the central masticatory pathways in patients with sleep bruxism. Neurosci Lett 2014;558:82–6.

75. Zhou WN, Fu HY, Du YF, et al. Short-term effects of repetitive transcranial magnetic stimulation on sleep bruxism—a pilot study. Int J Oral Sci 2016;8(1):61–5.

76. Cortes M, Black-Schaffer RM, Edwards DJ. Transcranial magnetic stimulation as an investigative tool for motor dysfunction and recovery in stroke: an overview for neurorehabilitation clinicians. Neuromodulation 2012;15(4):316–25.

77. Butler AJ, Kahn S, Wolf SL, et al. Finger extensor variability in TMS parameters among chronic stroke patients. J Neuroeng Rehabil 2005;2:10.

78. Groppa S, Oliviero A, Eisen A, et al. A practical guide to diagnostic transcranial magnetic stimulation: report of an IFCN committee. Clin Neurophysiol 2012;123(5):858–82.

79. Udupa K, Chen R. Central motor conduction time. Handb Clin Neurol 2013;116:375–86.

80. Turco CV, El-Sayes J, Savoie MJ, et al. Short- and long-latency afferent inhibition; uses, mechanisms and influencing factors. Brain Stimul 2018;11(1): 59–74.

81. Ziemann U, Rothwell JC, Ridding MC. Interaction between intracortical inhibition and facilitation in human motor cortex. J Physiol 1996;496(Pt 3):873–81.

82. Cui C, Song Y, Fan X, et al. Excitability of the masseter inhibitory reflex after high frequency rTMS over the motor cortex: a study in healthy humans. Arch Oral Biol 2017;82:241–6.

Statement of Ownership, Management, and Circulation
UNITED STATES POSTAL SERVICE® (All Periodicals Publications Except Requester Publications)

1. Publication Title	2. Publication Number	3. Filing Date
SLEEP MEDICINE CLINICS	025 – 053	9/18/2018

4. Issue Frequency	5. Number of Issues Published Annually	6. Annual Subscription Price
MAR, JUN, SEP, DEC	4	$203.00

7. Complete Mailing Address of Known Office of Publication (Not printer) (Street, city, county, state, and ZIP+4®)

ELSEVIER INC.
230 Park Avenue, Suite 800
New York, NY 10169

Contact Person
STEPHEN R. BUSHING

Telephone (Include area code)
215-239-3688

8. Complete Mailing Address of Headquarters or General Business Office of Publisher (Not printer)

ELSEVIER INC.
230 Park Avenue, Suite 800
New York, NY 10169

9. Full Names and Complete Mailing Addresses of Publisher, Editor, and Managing Editor (Do not leave blank)

Publisher (Name and complete mailing address)

TAYLORE BALL, ELSEVIER INC.
1600 JOHN F KENNEDY BLVD. SUITE 1800
PHILADELPHIA, PA 19103-2899

Editor (Name and complete mailing address)

COLLEEN DIETZLER, ELSEVIER INC.
1600 JOHN F KENNEDY BLVD. SUITE 1800
PHILADELPHIA, PA 19103-2899

Managing Editor (Name and complete mailing address)

PATRICK MANLEY, ELSEVIER INC.
1600 JOHN F KENNEDY BLVD. SUITE 1800
PHILADELPHIA, PA 19103-2899

10. Owner (Do not leave blank. If the publication is owned by a corporation, give the name and address of the corporation immediately followed by the names and addresses of all stockholders owning or holding 1 percent or more of the total amount of stock. If not owned by a corporation, give the names and addresses of the individual owners. If owned by a partnership or other unincorporated firm, give its name and address as well as those of each individual owner. If the publication is published by a nonprofit organization, give its name and address.)

Full Name	Complete Mailing Address
WHOLLY OWNED SUBSIDIARY OF REED/ELSEVIER, US HOLDINGS	1600 JOHN F KENNEDY BLVD. SUITE 1800 PHILADELPHIA, PA 19103-2899

11. Known Bondholders, Mortgagees, and Other Security Holders Owning or Holding 1 Percent or More of Total Amount of Bonds, Mortgages, or Other Securities. If none, check box ► ☐ None

Full Name	Complete Mailing Address
N/A	

12. Tax Status (For completion by nonprofit organizations authorized to mail at nonprofit rates) (Check one)
The purpose, function, and nonprofit status of this organization and the exempt status for federal income tax purposes:
☒ Has Not Changed During Preceding 12 Months
☐ Has Changed During Preceding 12 Months (Publisher must submit explanation of change with this statement)

PS Form 3526, July 2014 (Page 1 of 4 (see instructions page 4)) PSN: 7530-01-000-9931   PRIVACY NOTICE: See our privacy policy on www.usps.com.

---

13. Publication Title			14. Issue Date for Circulation Data Below
SLEEP MEDICINE CLINICS			JUNE 2018

15. Extent and Nature of Circulation			Average No. Copies Each Issue During Preceding 12 Months	No. Copies of Single Issue Published Nearest to Filing Date
a. Total Number of Copies (Net press run)			254	318
b. Paid Circulation (By Mail and Outside the Mail)	(1)	Mailed Outside-County Paid Subscriptions Stated on PS Form 3541 (Include paid distribution above nominal rate, advertiser's proof copies, and exchange copies)	165	193
	(2)	Mailed In-County Paid Subscriptions Stated on PS Form 3541 (Include paid distribution above nominal rate, advertiser's proof copies, and exchange copies)	0	0
	(3)	Paid Distribution Outside the Mails Including Sales Through Dealers and Carriers, Street Vendors, Counter Sales, and Other Paid Distribution Outside USPS®	30	41
	(4)	Paid Distribution by Other Classes of Mail Through the USPS (e.g., First-Class Mail®)	0	0
c. Total Paid Distribution (Sum of 15b (1), (2), (3), and (4))		►	195	234
d. Free or Nominal Rate Distribution (By Mail and Outside the Mail)	(1)	Free or Nominal Rate Outside-County Copies included on PS Form 3541	45	63
	(2)	Free or Nominal Rate In-County Copies included on PS Form 3541	0	0
	(3)	Free or Nominal Rate Copies Mailed at Other Classes Through the USPS (e.g., First-Class Mail)	0	0
	(4)	Free or Nominal Rate Distribution Outside the Mail (Carriers or other means)	0	0
e. Total Free or Nominal Rate Distribution (Sum of 15d (1), (2), (3) and (4))		►	45	63
f. Total Distribution (Sum of 15c and 15e)		►	240	297
g. Copies not Distributed (See Instructions to Publishers #4 (page #3))		►	14	21
h. Total (Sum of 15f and g)		►	254	318
i. Percent Paid (15c divided by 15f times 100)		►	81.25%	78.79%

* If you are claiming electronic copies, go to line 16 on page 3. If you are not claiming electronic copies, skip to line 17 on page 3.

16. Electronic Copy Circulation		Average No. Copies Each Issue During Preceding 12 Months	No. Copies of Single Issue Published Nearest to Filing Date
a. Paid Electronic Copies	►	0	0
b. Total Paid Print Copies (Line 15c) + Paid Electronic Copies (Line 16a)	►	195	234
c. Total Print Distribution (Line 15f) + Paid Electronic Copies (Line 16a)	►	240	297
d. Percent Paid (Both Print & Electronic Copies) (16b divided by 16c × 100)	►	81.25%	78.79%

☒ I certify that 50% of all my distributed copies (electronic and print) are paid above a nominal price.

17. Publication of Statement of Ownership

☒ If the publication is a general publication, publication of this statement is required. Will be printed
in the DECEMBER 2018 issue of this publication.

☐ Publication not required.

18. Signature and Title of Editor, Publisher, Business Manager, or Owner

[signature] Stephen R. Bushing

Date 9/18/2018

STEPHEN R. BUSHING – INVENTORY DISTRIBUTION CONTROL MANAGER

I certify that all information furnished on this form is true and complete. I understand that anyone who furnishes false or misleading information on this form or who omits material or information requested on the form may be subject to criminal sanctions (including fines and imprisonment) and/or civil sanctions (including civil penalties).

PS Form 3526, July 2014 (Page 3 of 4)   PRIVACY NOTICE: See our privacy policy on www.usps.com

Moving?

Make sure your subscription moves with you!

To notify us of your new address, find your **Clinics Account Number** (located on your mailing label above your name), and contact customer service at:

Email: journalscustomerservice-usa@elsevier.com

800-654-2452 (subscribers in the U.S. & Canada)
314-447-8871 (subscribers outside of the U.S. & Canada)

Fax number: 314-447-8029

Elsevier Health Sciences Division
Subscription Customer Service
3251 Riverport Lane
Maryland Heights, MO 63043

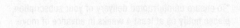